Clinical Cases
in Dermatolo

Series Editor
Robert A. Norman

For further volumes:
http://www.springer.com/series/10473

Dédée F. Murrell
Editor

Clinical Cases in Autoimmune Blistering Diseases

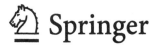 Springer

Editor
Dédée F. Murrell, M.A., BMBCh,
M.D., FAAD, FACD, FRCP
Department of Dermatology,
St George Hospital,
University of New South Wales
Kogarah, Sydney,
New South Wales
Australia

ISBN 978-3-319-10147-7   ISBN 978-3-319-10148-4   (eBook)
DOI 10.1007/978-3-319-10148-4
Springer Cham Heidelberg New York Dordrecht London

Library of Congress Control Number: 2014952791

Printed on acid-free paper

Springer is part of Springer Science+Business Media (www.springer.com)

Contents

Editors and Contributors

Editor

Dédée F. Murrell, M.A., BMBCh, M.D., FAAD, FACD, FRCP Department of Dermatology, St George Hospital Sydney, NSW, Australia

University of New South Wales, Sydney, NSW, Australia

Contributors

Valeria Aoki, M.D., Ph.D. Immunodermatology Laboratory, Department of Dermatology, University of Sao Paulo Medical School, São Paulo, Brazil

Kamran Balighi, M.D. Department of Dermatology, Autoimmune Bullous Research Centre, Razi Hospital, Tehran University of Medical Sciences, Tehran, Iran

Luca Borradori, M.D. Department of Dermatology, University Hospital Bern, Bern, Switzerland

Cheyda Chams-Davatchi, M.D. Department of Dermatology, Autoimmune Bullous Diseases Research Center, Tehran University of Medical Sciences, Tehran, Iran

Amy Y-Y Chen, M.D., FAAD Department of Dermatology, Boston University School of Medicine, Boston, MA, USA

Donna Aline Culton, M.D., Ph.D. Department of Dermatology, University of North Carolina at Chapel Hill, Chapel Hill, NC, USA

Maryam Daneshpazhooh, M.D. Department of Dermatology, Autoimmune Bullous Diseases Research Center, Tehran University of Medical Sciences, Tehran, Iran

Luis A. Diaz Department of Dermatology, University of North Carolina at Chapel Hill, Chapel Hill, NC, USA

Melanie Joy C. Doria University of New South Wales, Sydney, NSW, Australia

Department of Dermatology, St George Hospital, Sydney, NSW, Australia

David Fivenson, M.D. Department of Dermatology, PLLC, Ann Arbor, MI, USA

Maryam Ghiasi, M.D. Department of Dermatology, Autoimmune Bullous Diseases Research Center, Tehran University of Medical Sciences, Tehran, Iran

Autoimmune Bullous Diseases Research Center, Razi Hospital, Tehran, Iran

Adam G. Harris, MBChB Department of Dermatology, St George Hospital, Sydney, NSW, Australia

Stefanie Häfliger, M.D. Department of Dermatology, University Hospital Bern, Bern, Switzerland

Sarolta Kárpáti Department of Dermatology, Venereology and Dermatooncology, Semmelweis University, Budapest, Hungary

Monia Kharfi, M.D., Ph.D. Department of Dermatology, Hôpital Charles Nicolle, Tunis, Tunisia

Nokubonga F. Khoza, MBChB, FCDerm Department of Dermatology, Nelson R Mandela School of Medicine, University of Kwazulu-Natal, Durban, South Africa

Vahide Lajevardi, M.D. Autoimmune Bullous Diseases Research Center, Department of Dermatology, Tehran University of Medical Sciences, Tehran, Iran

Julia S. Lehman, M.D., FAAD Departments of Dermatology and Laboratory Medicine and Pathology, Mayo Clinic, Rochester, MN, USA

Nigel G. Maher, BMed, BDSc(Hons), B.Sc., FRACDS Department of Dermatology, St George Hospital, Sydney, NSW, Australia

University of New South Wales, Sydney, NSW, Australia

Denise Miyamoto, M.D. Immunodermatology Laboratory, Department of Dermatology, University of Sao Paulo Medical School, São Paulo, Brazil

Nayera H. Moftah, M.D. Department of Dermatology and Venereology, Faculty of Medicine for Girls, Al-Azhar University, Cairo, Egypt

Sophie-Charlotte Mook Department of Dermatology, University of Lübeck, Lübeck, Germany

Anisa Mosam, MBChB, FCDerm, MMed Department of Dermatology, Nelson R Mandela School of Medicine, University of Kwazulu-Natal, Durban, South Africa

Ziba Rahbar Autoimmune Bullous Diseases Research Center, Department of Dermatology, Tehran University of Medical Sciences, Tehran, Iran

Elizabeth S. Robinson, BSE Philadelphia Veteran Affairs Medical Center, Philadelphia, PA, USA

Department of Dermatology, University of Pennsylvania, Philadelphia, PA, USA

Zahra Safaei-Naraghi, M.D. Department of Dermatopathology, Autoimmune Bullous Research Centre, Razi Hospital, Tehran University of Medical Sciences, Tehran, Iran

Enno Schmidt, M.D., Ph.D. Department of Dermatology, University of Lübeck, Lübeck, Germany

Nina Schumacher Department of Dermatology, University of Lübeck, Lübeck, Germany

Iakov Shimanovich Department of Dermatology, University of Lübeck, Lübeck, Germany

Nina van Beek Department of Dermatology, University of Luebeck, Luebeck, Germany

Victoria P. Werth, M.D. Philadelphia Veteran Affairs Medical Center, Philadelphia, PA, USA

Department of Dermatology, University of Pennsylvania, Philadelphia, PA, USA

Kristen Whitney, DO Department of Dermatology, St Joseph Mercy Health System, Ann Arbor, MI, USA

Xinyi Yang University of New South Wales, Sydney, NSW, Australia

Cathy Zhao, M.B.B.S., MMed Department of Dermatology, St George Hospital, Sydney, NSW, Australia

Detlef Zillikens Department of Dermatology, University of Lübeck, Lübeck, Germany

Chapter 1
An Elderly Patient with a Generalized Pruritic Eruption

Stefanie Häfliger and Luca Borradori

A 86-year-old patient presented with generalized pruritic eruption of 3 month duration. The patient had a past history of type 2 insulin-dependent diabetes mellitus, dyslipidemia and arterial hypertension. On examination, the patient showed widespread excoriations, prurigo-like lesions, post-inflammatory hypopigmentations, with atrophic scarring distributed predominantly over his trunk, upper limbs, neck, and scalp (Fig. 1.1a–c). On his lower limbs, some scratched lesions were also observed. The patient also had isolated erosions on his buccal mucosa (Fig. 1.1d). Light microscopy studies showed changes consistent with chronic prurigo. Direct immunofluorescence microscopy studies obtained from perilesional skin showed linear deposits of IgG and C3 along the epidermal basement membrane zone. By indirect IF microscopy using NaCl-separated normal human skin, there were circulating IgG autoantibodies binding the epidermal side of the split. The search of circulating anti-BP180 antibodies by ELISA was positive (41.7 U/ml; N: $9 < $ U/ml).

S. Häfliger, M.D. • L. Borradori, M.D. (✉)
Department of Dermatology, University Hospital Bern, Freiburgstrasse, 3010 Bern, Switzerland
e-mail: Luca.Borradori@insel.ch and Stefanie.Haefliger@insel.ch

D.F. Murrell (ed.), *Clinical Cases in Autoimmune Blistering Diseases*, Clinical Cases in Dermatology 5, DOI 10.1007/978-3-319-10148-4_1,
© Springer International Publishing Switzerland 2015

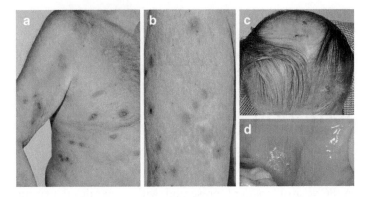

FIGURE 1.1 (**a**) Excoriations, postinflammatory hypopigmentations and atrophic scarring on trunk and arms; (**b**) Close-up view of excoriated lesions and scarring with isolated milia on arm; (**c**) Erosions, crusting and atrophic scarring on the scalp; (**d**) Erosion on buccal mucosa

What Is Your Diagnosis?

- Bullous pemphigoid (BP)
- Mucous membrane pemphigoid
- Brunsting-Perry pemphigoid

Discussion (1)

Diagnosis of BP is not always easy and straightforward. Manifestations of BP might resemble those of a variety of dermatoses, including drug reactions, contact dermatitis, prurigo, fixed urticaria, vasculitis, arthropod reaction and scabies (Table 1.1). Although the recent availability of ELISAs have facilitated the search of circulating autoantibodies, diagnosis still relies on a combination of clinical, histopathological and immunopathological features, particularly direct IF microscopy findings [5].

Our patient presented with chronic excoriated lesions and post-inflammatory changes predominantly localized on the

TABLE I.I   Clinical presentations of bullous pemphigoid

Chronic prurigo, prurigo nodularis-like features
Papular pemphigoid
Eczematous lesions
Erythema multiforme-like and Lyell-like pemphigoid
Lymphomatoid papulosis-like
Ecthyma-like
Palmo-plantar lesions (dysidrosiform pemphigoid)
Intertrigo (vegetating pemphigoid)
Vesicular pemphigoid
Erythrodermic pemphigoid
Brunsting-Perry form (variant of cicatricial pemphigoid with skin lesions)
Localized forms
Pretibial
Peristomal
Umbilical
"Stump" pemphigoid
On paralyzed body sites
On irradiated/traumatised body sites

upper trunk and his head and as well as isolated lesions of the buccal mucosa. Immunopathological findings were consistent with the pemphigoid group of autoimmune bullous disorders. We favor the diagnosis of an unusual form of chronic prurigo-like BP [5]. Nevertheless, our case presented also with features of the so called Brunsting-Perry variant of mucous membrane pemphigoid [2] with a peculiar extensive cutaneous involvement. In the absence of well recognized criteria, a conclusive classification of our case is not possible.

How Do You Manage This Patient?

- Topical corticosteroids
- Tetracyclines and nicotinamide
- Systemic steroids
- Systemic Steroids and immunsuppressants

Our BP patient was first treated with topical clobetasol propionate 0.05 % combined with doxyciclin, 200 mg daily and nicotinamide, 2 g daily. Since this regimen did not sufficiently control his skin disease, the patient was first given sulfasalazine and later oral prednisolone, 0.5 mg per kg body weight. The latter treatment resulted in control of the disease, but lead to a severe weight gain and a decompensation of his diabetes. Finally, topical steroids were initiated in combination with azathioprine 75 mg daily which lead to a complete remission of the skin disease.

Discussion (2)

BP has frequently a chronic evolution with remissions and relapses. It is associated with significant morbidity, such as severe itch, bullous and eroded lesions, and impetiginisation. The impact on the quality of life is significant [5].

Prior starting a therapy in patients with bullous pemphigoid, the overall clinical context and the evidence about the available therapeutic intervention should be considered: (1) affected patients have usually an advanced age, older than 75 years of age, (2) they have frequently additional comorbidities, such as neurological or cardiovascular diseases (3) they show a significantly increased mortality patients during the first year of treatment. Finally, (4) so far, except for topical and systemic steroids, there are no studies which have validated the use of the other drugs, which have been commonly used in BP [1].

The first line therapeutic option in localized, mild bullous pemphigoid consists of high potency topical corticosteroids based on their effectiveness demonstrated in two prospective controlled studies [3, 4].

Second-step and non-validated options include tetracyclines in combination with nicotinamide, topical calcineurin inhibitors and dapsone. Oral prednisone (0.5 mg/kg) can also be employed. In generalized disease, first-line treatment consist of either topical steroids applied to the entire body over 4–12 months [4] or of systemic corticosteroids (prednisolone, 0.5 mg/kg up to 1 mg/kg). The latter are effective, but result in more severe side effects and increased mortality. Immunosuppressants such as azathioprine, mycophenolate mofetil, methotrexate, chlorambucil can be used as second-step options in presence of contraindication to oral corticosteroids, corticosteroid-related complications and treatment-resistance. Controlled studies are needed to better define their place in management of BP as well as in preventing relapses of BP during the disease course. Finally, anecdotal cases of BP treated by rituximab (anti-CD20 antibody), omalizumab (anti-IgE antibody), plasma exchange, and intravenous immunoglobulins have also been described [1].

The optimal duration of treatment has not been defined. Based on clinical experience, we recommend an average treatment duration of 6–12 months, except in cases of steroid-resistance or steroid-dependence. The patients should be free of symptoms for 1 to 6 months under minimal therapy with oral prednisone (0.1 mg/kg/day), or clobetasol propionate (20 g/week), or immunosuppressants.

References

1. Daniel BS, Borradori L, Hall 3rd RP, Murrell DF. Evidence-based management of bullous pemphigoid. Dermatol Clin. 2011;29:613–20.
2. Hanno R, Foster DR, Bean SF. Brunsting-Perry cicatricial pemphigoid associated with bullous pemphigoid. J Am Acad Dermatol. 1980;3:470–3.
3. Joly P, Roujeau JC, Benichou J, Picard C, Dreno B, Delaporte E, Vaillant L, D'Incan M, Plantin P, Bedane C, Young P, Bernard P,

Bullous Diseases French Study Group. A comparison of oral and topical corticosteroids in patients with bullous pemphigoid. N Engl J Med. 2002;346:321–7.

4. Joly P, Roujeau JC, Benichou J, Delaporte E, D'Incan M, Dreno B, Bedane C, Sparsa A, Gorin I, Picard C, Tancrede-Bohin E, Sassolas B, Lok C, Guillaume JC, Doutre MS, Richard MA, Caux F, Prost C, Plantin P, Chosidow O, Pauwels C, Maillard H, Saiag P, Descamps V, Chevrant-Breton J, Dereure O, Hellot MF, Esteve E, Bernard P. A comparison of two regimens of topical corticosteroids in the treatment of patients with bullous pemphigoid: a multicenter randomized study. J Investig Dermatol. 2009;129:1681–7.

5. Schmidt E, della Torre R, Borradori L. Clinical features and practical diagnosis of bullous pemphigoid. Immunol Allergy Clin N Am. 2012;32:217–32.

Chapter 2
Confusion and Corticosteroids: 80-Year Old Woman with Pruritic Urticarial Plaques and Tense Blisters

Julia S. Lehman

An 80-year old woman with adult-onset diabetes mellitus presented to dermatology clinic several years ago with a 12-month history of a pruritic urticarial skin eruption of the flank and extremities. Her visit to dermatology was prompted by the new development of superimposed tense blisters (Fig. 2.1). She denied symptoms to suggest oropharyngeal, conjunctival, or genital mucosal involvement. Skin biopsy of perilesional skin demonstrated a subepidermal separation with eosinophilic spongiosis. Direct immunofluorescence showed linear deposition of C3 only. Indirect immunofluorescence with human salt-split skin showed linear deposition of IgG on the epidermal side of the blister. Enzyme-linked immunosorbent assay for BP180 and BP230 were elevated at 34 and 73 units, respectively (normal: <9 units).

Her clinical presentation, coupled with microscopic and immunologic data, supported a diagnosis of bullous pemphigoid (BP). Suffering from degenerative joint disease and

J.S. Lehman, M.D., FAAD
Departments of Dermatology and Laboratory Medicine and Pathology, Mayo Clinic, Rochester, MN, USA
e-mail: Lehman.Julia@mayo.edu

D.F. Murrell (ed.), *Clinical Cases in Autoimmune Blistering Diseases*, Clinical Cases in Dermatology 5, DOI 10.1007/978-3-319-10148-4_2, © Springer International Publishing Switzerland 2015

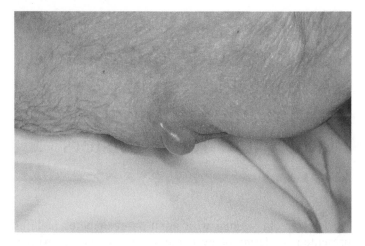

FIGURE 2.1 Tense inflammatory blister in a patient with bullous pemphigoid

living independently, the patient felt unable to apply topical corticosteroids, particularly given the widespread distribution of her lesions. Therefore, she was started on prednisone 1 mg/kg/day and mycophenolate mofetil. Being intolerant of the latter medication, she was then started on minocycline and niacinamide in lieu. In anticipation of long-term corticosteroid use, she was counseled by her dermatologist and primary care physician to take supplemental calcium, vitamin D, a bisphosphonate, trimethoprim-sulfamethoxazole for *Pneumocystis jiroveci* pneumonia (PCP) prophylaxis, and a proton-pump inhibitor. Given her comorbid diabetes mellitus, she was also advised to check her blood glucose levels frequently. After 3 weeks of immunosuppressive therapy, she reported marked improvement in her BP. Over the ensuing weeks, her prednisone dose was tapered.

Three months later, a flare of her BP prompted an increase of her prednisone dose back to 1 mg/kg/day. Shortly thereafter, she presented to the emergency department with altered mental status. Urinalysis showed elevated urinary ketones and glucose without bacteria, leukocyte esterase, or nitrites.

The most likely diagnosis is:

(A) Acute-onset of Alzheimer dementia, a neurologic condition associated with bullous pemphigoid
(B) Progressive multifocal leukoencephalopathy, an opportunistic infection by the JC virus
(C) Urinary tract infection, a common cause of confusion in the elderly
(D) Hyperglycemia, exacerbated by the patient's recently increased prednisone dose

Diagnosis

Hyperosmolar hyperglycemia in the setting of systemic corticosteroid therapy for bullous pemphigoid

Discussion

The patient's serum glucose level was found to exceed 600 mg/dL, confirming a diagnosis of hyperosmolar hyperglycemia. Her family revealed that she had become confused since her prednisone dose had increased, and she had not been diligent about checking her serum glucose at home. Following hospitalization for medical stabilization, and after confirming a normal serum thiopurine methyltransferase level, she was started on azathioprine and her prednisone dose was tapered to 5 mg/day. She has done well after 2 years of follow-up.

Bullous pemphigoid is a common autoimmune blistering disease associated with the development of autoantibodies against BP180 and BP230 antigens of the basement membrane zone. Although considerable evidence supports the use of topical corticosteroids in this condition [1, 2], logistical barriers associated with applying topical medications to widespread areas of the body in this often elderly population may necessitate the use of systemic corticosteroids to achieve rapid disease control in patients with widespread disease [3].

Although this patient had received high-dose prednisone, the best available evidence indicates that higher dose regimens of systemic corticosteroids offer no therapeutic benefit over lower dose regimens [4, 5]. Exposure to systemic corticosteroids should be minimized given their adverse side effect profile. Specific risks associated with systemic corticosteroids include hyperglycemia, osteopenia, delirium, osteonecrosis of the hip, *Pneumocystis jiroveci* pneumonia and other opportunistic infections, cataracts, redistribution of body fat, myopathy, gastric ulcers, and striae [6, 7]. Caused by reactivation of the JC virus, progressive multifocal leukoencephalopathy has been anecdotally reported to occur with prednisone use [8] but is more frequently observed as a complication of rituximab or efalizumab. Since systemic corticosteroid therapy can be prolonged in patients with BP, it is necessary to regularly look for opportunities to lower the dose, to closely monitor blood glucose in patients with glucose intolerance or frank diabetes mellitus and to address bone health, gastric protection, and *Pneumocystis* prophylaxis.

References

1. Joly P, Roujeau JC, Benichou J, Picard C, Dreno B, Delaporte E, Vaillant L, D'Incan M, Plantin P, Bedane C, Young P, Bernard P, Bullous Diseases French Study Group. A comparison of oral and topical corticosteroids in patients with bullous pemphigoid. N Engl J Med. 2002;346(5):321–7.
2. Fichel F, Barbe C, Joly P, Bedane C, Vabres P, Truchetet F, Aubin F, Michel C, Jegou J, Grange F, Antonicelli F, Bernard P. Clinical and immunologic factors associated with bullous pemphigoid relapse during the first year of treatment: a multicenter, prospective study. JAMA Dermatol. 2014;150(1):25–33.
3. Daniel BS, Borradori L, Hall 3rd RP, Murrell DF. Evidence-based management of bullous pemphigoid. Dermatol Clin. 2011;29(4): 613–20.
4. Kirtschig G, Middleton P, Bennett C, Murrell DF, Wojnarowska F, Khumalo NP. Interventions for bullous pemphigoid. Cochrane Database Syst Rev. 2010;10:CD002292.

5. Morel P, Guillaume J. Treatment of bullous pemphigoid with prednisolone only: 0.75 mg/kg/day versus 1.25 mg/kg/day. A multicenter randomized study. Ann Dermatol Venereol. 1984; 111(10):925–8.
6. Spivey J, Nye AM. Bullous pemphigoid: corticosteroid treatment and adverse effects in long-term care patients. Consult Pharm. 2013;28(7):455–62.
7. Frew JW, Murrell DF. Corticosteroid use in autoimmune blistering diseases. Immunol Allergy Clin North Am. 2012;32(2): 283–94.
8. Rosenbloom MA, Uphoff DF. The association of progressive multifocal leukoencephalopathy and sarcoidosis. Chest. 1983; 83(3):572–5.

Chapter 3
Bullous Pemphigoid and Tetracycline

Amy Y-Y. Chen

Case Presentation

An 85 year old female nursing home resident with a history of alcoholism, poorly controlled diabetes, hypertension and gout was brought to the dermatology clinic for a 6 month history of itchy skin and blisters. On exam, there were tense bullae on erythematous and normal appearing skin as well as urticarial, eroded and crusted plaques on the inner aspects of bilateral upper and lower extremities, and extensor surfaces of lower extremities (Fig. 3.1). Nikolsky's sign was negative and the oral mucosa was clear. Her current medications include hydrochlorothiazide, lisinopril, glipizide, metformin and allopurinol. Two biopsies were performed. H&E showed subepidermal bullae with numerous eosinophils and rare neutrophils. No acantholysis. Direct immunofluorescence demonstrates linear IgG and C3 along the basement membrane. A diagnosis of bullous pemphigoid was made. What is the best management option for her?

A.Y-Y. Chen, M.D., FAAD
Department of Dermatology, Boston University School of
Medicine, 609 Albany Street, J501, Boston, MA 02118, USA
e-mail: ayyen@alum.mit.edu

D.F. Murrell (ed.), *Clinical Cases in Autoimmune
Blistering Diseases*, Clinical Cases in Dermatology 5,
DOI 10.1007/978-3-319-10148-4_3,
© Springer International Publishing Switzerland 2015

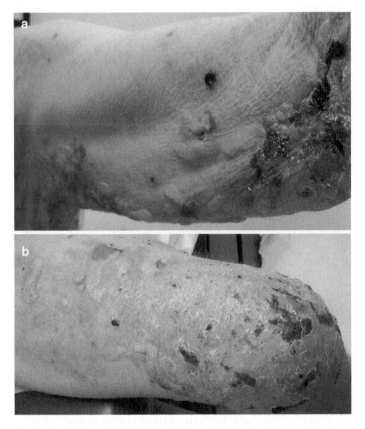

FIGURE 3.1 Tense bullae on erythematous and normal appearing skin as well as urticarial, eroded and crusted plaques on the inner aspects of bilateral upper arms (**a**) and extensor surfaces of lower extremities (**b**)

(A) Azathioprine
(B) Methotrexate
(C) Rituximab
(D) **Tetracycline and Nicotinamide**
(E) Prednisone

Discussion

Topical and systemic prednisone as well as other steroid sparing systemic immunosuppressive agents have traditionally been used in the treatment of bullous pemphigoid (BP). Since BP typically occurs in elderly patients with various other medical problems as well as co-morbidities, a steroid sparing agent with excellent safety profile is needed for management.

Tetracycline (TCN) was first reported as an effective treatment for BP in the 1980s, either alone or in combination with nicotinamide (niacinamide) [2, 16]. Since that time, many case reports and case series have demonstrated good response in treating both localized and generalized BP with TCN (Table 3.1) or one of its family members of antibiotics (Table 3.2), either alone or in combination with nicotinamide, with or without moderate to high potency topical steroids. The current discussion will focus on TCN, as it has been used most extensively in the treatment of BP.

The TCN family of antibiotics inhibits bacterial protein synthesis by binding to the 30S subunit of the bacterial ribosome. They are bacteriostatic. Currently available TCN family antibiotics include the short acting TCN (half-life 6–12 h), the intermediate acting demeclocycline (half-life 16 h), and the long acting doxycycline (half-life 18–22 h) and minocycline (half-life 11–22 h). Doxycycline and minocycline are well absorbed in the presence or absence of food, while TCN and demeclocycline are better absorbed in the fasting state. Unlike other TCN family antibiotics, which are metabolized renally, doxycycline is metabolized by the gastrointestinal tract and therefore is the only oral TCN family member acceptable for use in renal failure patients. Due to potential hepatotoxicity, TCN family antibiotics are relatively contraindicated in patients with severe liver disease [1].

In addition to its antimicrobial activities, TCNs also have anti-inflammatory properties. It is these anti-inflammatory properties of TCNs that have been postulated to play a role

TABLE 3.1 Summary of BP treated with TCN +/– Nicotinamide +/– topical steroids

Reference	TCN starting dose	Nicotinamide	Topical steroids	Other concomitant systemic therapy	# of patients	Results
Pereyo and Davis [13]	500 mg bid	N/A	N/A	N/A	1	All bullae and inflammatory lesions cleared in 2 weeks
Thornfeldt and Menkes [16][a]	250–500 mg bid	N/A	N/A	1 received systemic prednisone	2	Complete resolution in 3 weeks
Thomas et al. [15]	1–2 g daily in divided doses	N/A	Betamethasone valerate 0.1 % cream, betamethasone dipropionate 0.05 % cream and fluocinoide 0.05 % ointment	N/A	5	Re-epithelialization in 1–3 weeks. No blister at 1–3 weeks

Fivenson et al. [4]	500 mg qid	500 mg tid	N/A	N/A	12	During the initial 8 weeks period: 5 had complete response, 5 had partial response, 1 with no response and 1 with worsening of disease. TCN was changed to minocycline 100 mg bid in 2 patients due to side effects
Kolbach et al. [10]	2 g daily in divided doses	2 g daily in divided doses	N/A	3/7 received systemic prednisone	7	Blister formation significantly reduced within 1–2 weeks. Bullae ceased to develop in 6–8 weeks
Goon et al. [5]	1.5–2 g daily in divided doses	1.5–2 g daily in divided doses	Betamethasone valerate 0.05–0.1 % cream	N/A	5	4/5 on TCN had complete response, 1/5 had partial response

(continued)

TABLE 3.1 (continued)

Reference	TCN starting dose	Nicotinamide	Topical steroids	Other concomitant systemic therapy	# of patients	Results
Berk and Lorincz [2]	1–2 g daily in divided doses	1.5–2.5 g daily in divided doses	2/4 received 0.1 % triamcinolone acetonide ointment	1 also received dapsone	4	Responded within 1–2 weeks. 1 had occasional outbreak. 1 had recurrence and received erythromycin ethylsuccinate three times daily with good control; unclear why TCN was not reinitiated
Hornschuh et al. [7]	500 mg qid	400 mg bid	0.5 % clobetasol	N/A	16	Within 4 weeks, 13/16 had complete response, 2/16 did not respond

bid twice a day, *tid* three times a day, *qid* four times a day

[a]Localized BP; *N/A* not applicable

TABLE 3.2 Summary of BP treated with other TCN family antibiotics +/– Nicotinamide +/– topical steroids

Reference	Antibiotics starting dose	Nicotinamide	Topical steroids	Other concomitant systemic therapy	# of patients	Results
Safa and Darrieux [14][a]	Doxycycline bid	N/A	N/A	N/A	4	Pruritus resolved and complete clearance of skin lesions seen in 1–4 weeks
Goon et al. [5][b]	Doxycycline bid	Nicotinamide 1.5–2 g daily in divided doses	N/A	Prednisone in those with no response or progressive disease. 1 with progressive disease also got dapsone	6	2 with complete response, 1 with partial response, 1 with no response and 2 with progressive disease
Kakurai et al. [8]	Minocycline unclear dose	N/A	Yes unclear which	N/A	1	Lesions resolve in 7 weeks

(continued)

TABLE 3.2 (continued)

Reference	Antibiotics starting dose	Nicotinamide	Topical steroids	Other concomitant systemic therapy	# of patients	Results
Loo et al. [11]	Minocycline as adjuvant: 50 mg daily and increase to 100 mg bid if tolerated after 1–2 weeks	N/A	Yes in some with clobetasol propionate 0.05 %	Yes in majority (prednisolone, dapsone, methotrexate, cyclosporine, azathioprine)	22	6 with major response, 11 with minor response, 5 with no response. Introduction of minocycline reduced systemic prednisone requirement in those on it

bid twice a day

[a]Non bullous BP

[b]Received doxycycline (instead of TCN) due to inability to tolerate tetracycline, better compliance or other medical reasons

in its effectiveness in the treatment of BP. Along with IgG, IgE is often deposited in BP lesions. When mast cells are activated by IgE, pro-inflammatory cytokines attracting eosinophils and neutrophils are released. TCN has been shown to inhibit neutrophil and eosinophil chemotaxis, activation, and migration in both in vitro and in vivo studies [3, 4, 12]. In addition, neutrophil elastase has been implicated in the basement membrane (BM) destruction of BP. TCN indirectly inhibits neutrophil elastase, therefore preventing further destruction of the BM zone [12].

Nicotinamide, also known as niacinamide, is often used in combination with TCN and other members of its family of antibiotics in the treatment of BP (Tables 3.1 and 3.2). To the best of the author's knowledge, nicotinamide monotherapy has been reported only once as a successful treatment in a patient with localized BP [6]. Nicotinic acid (niacin, vitamin B3) is an essential dietary constituent. In the body, nicotinic acid is converted to nicotinamide [9]. Nicotinamide is relatively safe. Although potential side effects such as hepatotoxicity and pruritus could occur, these are rare events and have generally been reported in patients who are taking a much higher dose than that use to manage BP [4, 9]. In contrast to nicotinic acid, nicotinamide is not a vasodilator and flushing is typically not associated with it [9].

Nicotinamide functions as a crucial coenzyme that accepts hydrogen ions in oxidation-reduction reactions essential for tissue respiration [9]. Nicotinamide has not only been shown to block antigen-IgE-induced histamine release both in vitro and in vivo, but it has also been shown to prevent mast cell degranulation in sensitized guinea pig tissues [2]. Similar to TCN, nicotinamide inhibits neutrophil and eosinophil chemotaxis and secretion [4]. Therefore, its efficacy in BP may work partly by stabilizing the mast cell, prohibiting the release of eosinophilic chemotactic factor and other inflammatory mediators produced by complement activation [2]. Nicotinamide also has a potent inhibitory effect on serum phosphodiesterase, with resultant increase in cyclic adenosine monophosphate (cAMP). Increasing cAMP levels decrease the release of proteases from lymphocytes, further contributing to the anti-inflammatory effect of nicotinamide [9]. Nicotinamide may also exert its therapeutic function via electron scavenging and/or increased tryptophan conversion to serotonin [4].

In cases reports and case series published so far, the TCN doses for BP management range from 500 mg to 2 g daily in divided doses, and the nicotinamide doses range from 800 mg to 2.5 g daily in divided doses. Responses are usually seen within the first few weeks (Table 3.1). There has been no study comparing the combination of TCN plus nicotinamide with either therapy alone in the treatment of BP. It is likely that the anti-inflammatory effect of nicotinamide works synergistically with the anti-inflammatory effect of TCN [2, 4]. Once the skin disease is under control and clear, various tapering regimens have been proposed. One group of authors who started their patients with TCN 500 mg four times daily plus nicotinamide 400 mg three times a day suggest reducing the dose of TCN in decrements of 500 mg every 4 weeks down to 250 mg four times daily, and subsequently in steps of 250 mg every 4 weeks. Nicotinamide was reduced in steps of 600 mg every month [7]. Timing of tapering also differs among different authors, with some authors recommending waiting for a 6 month period before trial of gradual withdrawal of therapy [2].

In an 18 patient randomized, open-label trial comparing the combination of 500 mg of nicotinamide three times daily plus 500 mg of TCN four times daily with systemic prednisone treatment, the trial failed to show a statistically significant difference in reduction in numbers of skin lesions, responses for pruritus, or the physician's global assessment between the two groups. Twelve patients received a combination of TCN and nicotinamide and six received prednisone therapy. In the combination group, five achieved complete response, five achieved partial response, one had no response and one had worsening of the disease during the initial 8-week period. In the prednisone group, one reached complete response and five achieved partial response. Two patients in the combination group reported gastrointestinal upset, and TCN was changed to minocycline 100 mg twice daily. One patient with elevated baseline serum creatinine and serum urea nitrogen concentration developed acute tubular necrosis after 4 weeks of combination therapy. Return of baseline renal function was obtained 2 weeks after discontinuation of therapy. In contrast, there was one occurrence each of hypertension, erosive gastritis, multiple decubitus ulcers, osteomyelitis, deep venous thrombosis, and death related to sepsis in the prednisone group. Two prednisone-treated patients also required insulin therapy for hyperglycemia [4].

Although the only randomized, open label study discussed above comparing a combination of TCN plus nicotinamide and prednisone in BP did not show a statistically significant difference between the two groups in assessed parameters, in elderly patients with multiple comorbidities, the combination of TCN and nicotinamide appears to be a safe, reasonable and useful alternative to systemic steroid and/or other steroid sparing immunosuppressive therapy. Perhaps a larger randomized controlled trial comparing the combination of TCN and nicotinamide with systemic prednisone will demonstrate a statistical significance.

In those who cannot tolerate TCN or when TCN is contraindicated, despite a lack of strong evidence, substituting TCN with other antibiotics of the TCN family such as doxycycline or minocycline is a logical option, given their similar anti-inflammatory effect. Further studies comparing efficacy in the treatment of BP among the various members of the TCN family of antibiotics with and without nicotinamide will also be invaluable in providing evidence to support or refute their use in clinical practice.

Key Points

-   In elderly patients with BP and other comorbidities, the combination of TCN and nicotinamide appears to be a safe, reasonable and useful alternative to systemic steroid and/or other steroid sparing immunosuppressive therapy.

References

1. Ashourian N, Cohen P. Systemic antibacterial agents. In: Wolverton S, editor. Comprehensive dermatologic drug therapy. Philadelphia: Elsevier; 2007.
2. Berk MA, Lorincz AL. The treatment of bullous pemphigoid with tetracycline and niacinamide. A preliminary report. Arch Dermatol. 1986;122:670–4.
3. Esterly NB, Furey NL, Flanagan LE. The effect of antimicrobial agents on leukocyte chemotaxis. J Invest Dermatol. 1978;70:51–5.
4. Fivenson DP, Breneman DL, Rosen GB, Hersh CS, Cardone S, Mutasim D. Nicotinamide and tetracycline therapy of bullous pemphigoid. Arch Dermatol. 1994;130:753–8.
5. Goon AT, Tan SH, Khoo LS, Tan T. Tetracycline and nicotinamide for the treatment of bullous pemphigoid: our experience in Singapore. Singapore Med J. 2000;41:327–30.
6. Honl BA, Elston DM. Autoimmune bullous eruption localized to a breast reconstruction site: response to niacinamide. Cutis. 1998;62:85–6.
7. Hornschuh B, Hamm H, Wever S, Hashimoto T, Schroder U, Brocker EB, Zillikens D. Treatment of 16 patients with bullous pemphigoid with oral tetracycline and niacinamide and topical clobetasol. J Am Acad Dermatol. 1997;36:101–3.
8. Kakurai M, Demitsu T, Azuma R, Yamada T, Suzuki M, Yoneda K, Ishii N, Hashimoto T. Localized pemphigoid (pretibial type) with IgG antibody to BP180 NC16a domain successfully treated with minocycline and topical corticosteroid. Clin Exp Dermatol. 2007;32:759–61.
9. Knable AL, Davis LS. Miscellaneous systemic drugs. In: Wolverton S, editor. Comprehensive dermatologic drug therapy. Philadelphia: Elsevier; 2007.
10. Kolbach DN, Remme JJ, Bos WH, Jonkman MF, DE Jong MC, Pas HH, van der Meer JB. Bullous pemphigoid successfully controlled by tetracycline and nicotinamide. Br J Dermatol. 1995;133:88–90.
11. Loo WJ, Kirtschig G, Wojnarowska F. Minocycline as a therapeutic option in bullous pemphigoid. Clin Exp Dermatol. 2001;26:376–9.
12. Monk E, Shalita A, Siegel DM. Clinical applications of non-antimicrobial tetracyclines in dermatology. Pharmacol Res. 2011;63:130–45.

13. Pereyo NG, Davis LS. Generalized bullous pemphigoid controlled by tetracycline therapy alone. J Am Acad Dermatol. 1995;32:138–9.
14. Safa G, Darrieux L. Nonbullous pemphigoid treated with doxycycline monotherapy: report of 4 cases. J Am Acad Dermatol. 2011;64:e116–8.
15. Thomas I, Khorenian S, Arbesfeld DM. Treatment of generalized bullous pemphigoid with oral tetracycline. J Am Acad Dermatol. 1993;28:74–7.
16. Thornfeldt CR, Menkes AW. Bullous pemphigoid controlled by tetracycline. J Am Acad Dermatol. 1987;16:305–10.

Chapter 4
A 52-Year-Old Italian Male with Widespread Blistering and Erosions Refractory to Regular Dose Prednisone

Nigel G. Maher and Dédée F. Murrell

A 52 year-old Australian male of Italian descent began experiencing blisters and erosions on his trunk, face, scalp and mouth in November 2002. Skin biopsy revealed an intraepidermal suprabasal split, and on direct immunofluorescence, IgG and C3 were positive intercellularly in the epidermis. He was admitted to hospital and commenced on 25 mg prednisolone. He discharged himself against medical advice and represented at our centre 4 months later in pain with widespread erosions and crusting on his face, scalp, chest, back and mouth, along with hypertension with a blood pressure of 148/118 (Fig. 4.1).

His co-morbidities included hypertension, hyperlipidemia, hypertriglyceridemia, obstructive sleep apnoea, gastro-oesophageal reflux, and lactose intolerance. In addition, his previous medical history included infection with herpes

N.G. Maher, BMed, BDSc(Hons), B.Sc., FRACDS
D.F. Murrell, M.A., BMBCh, M.D., FAAD, FACD (✉)
Department of Dermatology, St George Hospital,
Gray St, Kogarah, Sydney, NSW 2217, Australia

University of New South Wales, Sydney, NSW Australia
e-mail: d.murrell@unsw.edu.au

D.F. Murrell (ed.), *Clinical Cases in Autoimmune Blistering Diseases*, Clinical Cases in Dermatology 5, DOI 10.1007/978-3-319-10148-4_4,
© Springer International Publishing Switzerland 2015

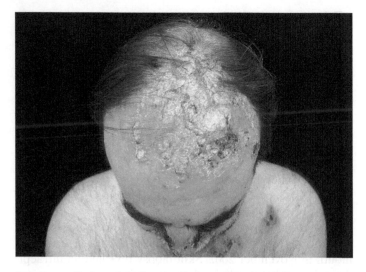

FIGURE 4.1 Scalp at initial presentation in March 2003

simplex type 2 and syphilis, an episode of viral pericarditis, recurrent bladder infections, and an appendicectomy.

His medications at the time of first assessment were: prednisolone (25 mg daily), omeprazole, lisinopril, frusemide, aldactone, a multivitamin and L-lysine.

Based on the clinical history and biopsy findings, what is your most likely diagnosis from the options below?

1. Mucous membrane pemphigoid
2. Bullous pemphigoid
3. Linear IgA dermatosis
4. Pemphigus vulgaris
5. Bullous lupus erythematous

Diagnosis

Pemphigus Vulgaris

Further indirect immunofluorescence studies in April 2003 on monkey oesophagus, showed intercellular positivity for

IgG. Desmolgein ELISA was not available at that time in Australia.

As he had already been commenced on prednisolone for 4 months, he had a baseline DEXA scan, which was normal. Nonetheless, he was also commenced on alendronate, calcium and vitamin D supplements due to the risk of osteoporosis caused by steroid treatment.

For treatment of his pemphigus vulgaris (PV), he was commenced on prednisolone 1 mg/kg/day, and azathioprine 50 mg daily initially. However, after several weeks of treatment with this regime, his skin lesions caused by PV became worse and he was experiencing intense pain. He was admitted to hospital and had daily baths, the azathioprine was ceased, and he was commenced on mycophenolate mofetil at 750 mg twice a day, and the prednisolone was increased to 100 mg twice a day. For his pain he was started on paracetamol and tramadol, but the tramadol was later ceased due to side effects and amitriptyline was introduced as an adjunct with paracetamol. Due to the high doses of prednisolone required to bring his disease under control, he became Cushingoid, and experienced severe mood swings and mania (which resulted in a large credit card debt). He was referred to a psychiatrist, who managed this with citalopram.

His PV eventually stabilized after 3 weeks in hospital and by May 2003 the prednisolone started to be weaned. He was noted to have slowly healing persistent lesions, which was treated with topical mometasone furoate 0.1 %. His prednisolone was gradually tapered over the following 4 months to 5 mg/day by November 2003, whence the alendronate was ceased (Fig. 4.2).

An indirect immunofluorescence serum titer on monkey oesophagus in January 2004 remained positive at 1:80. By March 2004 he was being maintained on 5 mg of prednisolone and mycophenolate mofetil 1,000 mg twice a day.

He had a persistent scalp erosion that was managed with betamethasone dipropionate 0.05 %, and triamcinalone (5 mg/cc) injections. By April 2005, the scalp lesion had completely healed, only for it to flare again in June 2005. This time, mometasone furoate 0.1 % solution along with a tar and salicyclic acid preparation was used to treat the scalp.

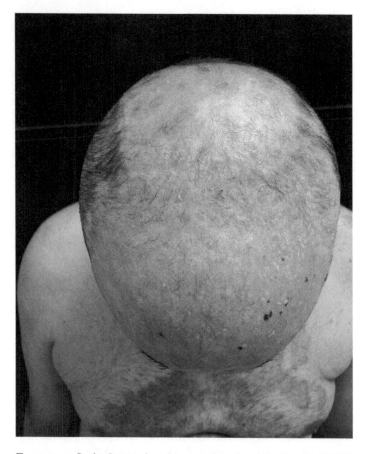

FIGURE 4.2 Scalp 9 months after commencement of treatment in January 2004

The prednisolone was finally discontinued in August 2006, with a stable disease state, and persistent erosions on the scalp and nose, and intermittently in the mouth. Mycophenolate mofetil was continued at 1,000 mg twice a day, a dexamethasone 2 mg mouthrinse was used to control the oral erosions, and mometasone furoate 0.1 % lotion was used topically to affected cutaneous sites twice a day.

Over the next 5 years, the mycophenolate mofetil was gradually titrated down to 250 mg twice a week. Follow-up indirect immunofluorescence in February 2011 revealed no circulating IgG and IgA autoantibodies detected on monkey oesophagus nor human salt split skin. ELISAs with recombinant desmoglein 1 and 3 antibodies were negative (<2 U/mL). This indicated no serological evidence of PV and the mycophenolate mofetil was finally ceased, such that he was in complete remission off therapy.

Discussion

PV is an autoimmune, acquired condition, that has a female preponderance and prevalent onset in the fifth decade of life [1, 2]. Evidence has linked the pathophysiology to autoantibodies against keratinocyte antigens desmoglein 3 and desmoglein 1, with a mucosal disease phenotype most commonly associated with autoantibodies to desmoglein 3, and a cutaneous phenotype associated with autoantibodies to desmoglein 1 [3, 4]. This phenotypic pattern was attributed to the anatomic differences in desmoglein 1 and 3 distribution between the cutaneous and mucosal epithelium. However, more recent evidence has suggested the pathophysiology in PV involves a more complex interplay between other antigens and non-desmoglein antibodies [5, 6]. Furthermore, the autoantibody titers against desmoglein 1 and 3 have been shown not to match the predicted phenotypic patterns [6]. Nonetheless, anti-desmoglein 1 and 3 antibody titers from an ELISA are still useful to guide treatment. However, it must be also be remembered that when treatment is commenced, the clinical manifestations of PV will improve earlier than these antibody titers [6]. This patient was unusual in that he had predominantly a cutaneous only phenotype with later onset of more oral mucosal involvement, and his desmoglein 1 and 3 ELISAs were negative, albeit later in the disease course.

Systemic corticosteroid therapy, at moderate to high doses, is typically necessary to acutely control the disease at onset. Moderate doses are regarded as 1 mg/kg/day oral prednisone [6]. In milder disease, starting doses of 40–60 mg prednisone per day have been suggested, while in more severe disease, starting doses of 60–100 mg per day may be advisable [7]. These doses may be need to be increased by 50–100 % each week should there be no response [7]. When doses greater than 100 mg per day of prednisone are required, then pulsed intravenous corticosteroid may be an alternative.

In this patient, a very low starting dose of prednisone was initiated by another dermatologist, and failed to bring the disease under control. Escalation of therapy was quickly required to bring the disease under control, and hence the prednisone dose was increased to 100 mg twice a day. In addition, adjunctive therapy was initiated – initially as azathioprine, and then to mycophenolate as the disease continued to progress. The problem with adjunctive therapies is their latency time to clinical improvement. Azathioprine has a latency time of at least 6 weeks before clinical efficacy is observed [7]. Mycophenolate has been shown to have efficacy within 8 weeks [8] although longer treatment is necessary to induce remission [9].

Adjunctive drug therapies for PV can include azathioprine, cyclophosphamide, mycophenolate, gold, nicotinamide, tetracyclines, TNF-alpha antagonists and rituximab [6, 7, 10]. The most common adjunctive therapies for PV are azathioprine and cyclophosphamide, although mycophenolate is gaining popularity due to the perceived better side-effect profile compared to some other agents [9]. Adjunctive therapies have an important role in long term disease control and achieving remission, particularly given the wide range of comorbidities induced by long term corticosteroid use, although so far only one randomized controlled trial of pooled data has been able to show this [11].

In the example patient, the high dose steroids needed to control his PV resulted in psychiatric symptoms (mania, mood swings), difficulty sleeping, acne vulgaris and Cushingoid features. In addition, he required close monitoring for osteoporosis and diabetes mellitus – for which he was referred to an endocrinologist. Other side effects of corticosteroids include hypertension, hypothalamic-pituitary-adrenal suppression, menstrual disorders, hyperlipidemia, atherosclerosis, cardiovascular events, fatty liver, cataracts, glaucoma, pseudotumor cerebri, pancreatitis, growth retardation, osteonecrosis, myopathy, muscle cramps and weakness, skin bruising and atrophy, and peptic ulcer disease [6]. The clinician must bear in mind these co-morbidities when using corticosteroids, particularly at high doses for prolonged periods.

With mycophenolate, it also important to remember that higher doses (35–45 mg/kg/day) are typically required to treat immunobullous disorders compared to the doses used in renal transplant patients (30 mg/kg/day) [9]. This is because of the additional agents used in renal transplant agents such as cyclosporin or tacrolimus [9]. The most common side effect of mycophenolate is mild gastrointestinal distress [9], which the patient in this example experienced with a sensation of abdominal bloating.

Other adjunctive therapies, such as intravenous immunoglobulin, plasma exchange and extracorporeal photopheresis may also be considered in cases where PV is refractory to conventional drug therapies, or the side-effects of the medication are a significant concern [7].

Key Pearls

PV can sometimes require high doses of corticosteroids for prolonged periods to bring the disease under control.

Careful monitoring for side effects of corticosteroid therapy should take place, and multi-disciplinary treatment may be warranted. Steroid-sparing drugs can help to reduce the exposure to systemic steroids.

References

1. Gupta V, Kelbel T, Nguyen D, Melonakos K, Murrell D, Xie Y, et al. A globally available internet-based patient survey of pemphigus vulgaris: epidemiology and disease characteristics. Dermatol Clin. 2011;29(3):393–404.
2. Venugopal S, Murrell D. Diagnosis and clinical features of pemphigus vulgaris. Dermatol Clin. 2011;29(3):373–80.

3. Amagai M, Koch P, Nishikawa T, Stanley J. Pemphigus vulgaris antigen (desmoglein 3) is localized in the lower epidermis, the site of blister formation in patients. J Invest Dermatol. 1996;106(2):351–5.
4. Ding X, Diaz L, Fairley J, Giudice G, Liu Z. The anti-desmoglein 1 autoantibodies in pemphigus vulgaris sera are pathogenic. J Invest Dermatol. 1999;112(5):739–43.
5. Chernyavsky A, Arrendondo J, Kitajima Y, Sato-Nagai M, Grando S. Desmoglein versus non-desmoglein signaling in pemphigus acantholysis: characterization of novel signaling pathways downstream of pemphigus vulgaris antigens. J Biol Chem. 2007;282(18):13804–12.
6. Grando S. Pemphigus autoimmunity: hypotheses and realities. Autoimmunity. 2011;45(1):7–35.
7. Harman K, Albert S, Black M. Guidelines for the management of pemphigus vulgaris. Br J Dermatol. 2003;149(5):926–37.
8. Enk A, Knop J. Mycophenolate is effective in the treatment of pemphigus vulgaris. Arch Dermatol. 1999;135(1):54–6.
9. Mimouni D, Anhalt G, Cummins D, Kouba D, Thorne J, Nousari C. Treatment of pemphigus vulgaris and pemphigus foliaceus with mycophenolate mofetil. Arch Dermatol. 2003;139(6):739–42.
10. Daniel B, Murrell D, Joly P. Rituximab and its use in autoimmune bullous disorders. Dermatol Clin. 2011;29(4):571–5.
11. Chams-Davatchi C, Esmaili N, Daneshpazhooh M, Valikhani M, Balighi K, Hallaji Z, et al. Randomized controlled open-label trial of four treatment regimens for pemphigus vulgaris. J Am Acad Dermatol. 2007;57(4):622–8.

Chapter 5
Life-Threatening Pemphigus Vulgaris

Nina Schumacher, Sophie-Charlotte Mook, Iakov Shimanovich, Detlef Zillikens, and Enno Schmidt

A 69-year-old male was transferred to our department by helicopter on a Sunday morning from the intensive care burn unit of another university hospital. In this unit, he had been treated for 3 days including a radical debridement of unattached skin. Before, he had been admitted in a dermatology department of another university hospital for exacerbated pemphigus vulgaris. Pemphigus had been diagnosed 2 years ago and treated with tapering doses of initially high-dose oral corticosteroids and mycophenolate mofetil before dramatic worsening of oral and skin lesions 3 months ago with a weight loss of 25 kg and generalized erosions and blistering. At the time of presentation in our clinic due to his poor general condition his only immunosuppressive medication was mycophenolate mofetil at a dose of 1 g/day.

What is the most relevant differential diagnosis in this patient?

1. Bullous drug eruption
2. Paraneoplastic pemphigus

N. Schumacher • S.-C. Mook • I. Shimanovich
D. Zillikens • E. Schmidt, M.D., Ph.D. (✉)
Department of Dermatology, University of Lübeck,
Ratzeburger Allee 160, D-23538 Lübeck, Germany
e-mail: enno.schmidt@uksh.de

D.F. Murrell (ed.), *Clinical Cases in Autoimmune Blistering Diseases*, Clinical Cases in Dermatology 5, DOI 10.1007/978-3-319-10148-4_5,
© Springer International Publishing Switzerland 2015

3. Bullous pemphigoid
4. Staphylococcal scalded skin syndrome
5. Mucous membrane pemphigoid

On examination, extensive erosions involving the buccal mucosa, tongue, and hard and soft palate with pseudomembrane formation were seen. In addition, crusted erosions were present on the lips and hemorrhagic crusts on the nasal mucosa. Erosions and flaccid blisters affected more than 70 % of body surface area (Fig. 5.1). The pemphigus disease area index (PDAI) [1] was 220. Laboratory investigations demonstrated high levels of circulating antibodies against desmoglein 1 (1,045 U/ml) and desmoglein 3 (3,572 U/ml) as detected by ELISA (Euroimmun, Lübeck, Germany).

Due to poor general condition, severe stomatitis and involvement of lips paraneoplastic pemphigus was excluded by indirect immunofluorescence on rat and monkey bladder, immunoblotting with extract from cultured keratinocytes (containing full length periplakin, envoplakin, and desmoplakin I/II), and envoplakin ELISA (Euroimmun) [2].

The patient was in a reduced general condition with signs of systemic illness including tachycardia and hypotension, for what he received noradrenalin infusions. After 2 days on the Intensive Care Unit (ICU), we initiated a combination treatment with immunoadsorption on three consecutive days (1 cycle) and an i.v. dexamethasone pulse (100 mg/day for three consecutive days) followed by high-dose i.v. immunoglobulins (IVIG; 2 g/kg of body weight) and an increase of the mycophenolate mofetil dose to 2 g/day (Fig. 5.2). Daily wound care consisted of antiseptic (polihexanide or alginate hydrogel) and non-adhesive wound dressings. Due to the pain associated with oral food intake, parenteral nutrition was necessary to provide adequate nutritional support. In fact, dehydration, hypovolaemia and electrolyte abnormalities necessitated intravenous fluid replacement of up to 7 l per day. The patient was embedded in an air-fluidized temperature-controlled bed on laminated sheets and synthetic dressings. After no improvement of pemphigus lesions for 2 weeks, a single cyclophosphamide bolus (600 mg i.v.)

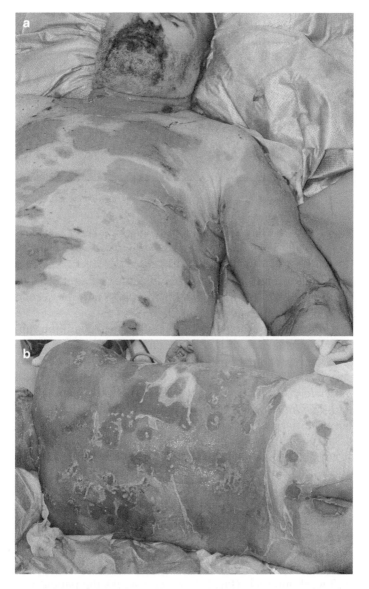

FIGURE 5.1 Extensive erosions on the dorsal trunk, buttocks proximal upper extremities (**a**) and chest (**b**) at first presentation in our department

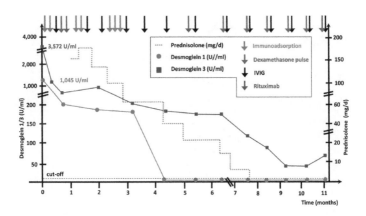

FIGURE 5.2 Schematic diagram of the treatment protocol and corresponding autoantibody serum levels during the course of the disease

was administered, rituximab treatment was initiated (four infusions of 375 mg/m^2 in weekly intervals) and the second cycle of immunoadsorption and IVIG was given.

Unfortunately, the patient's overall clinical condition rapidly deteriorated with high fever and increased CRP serum levels necessitating transfer to the ICU for cardio-respiratory support. The patient developed septic shock, with *Staphyloccocus aureus*, *Acinetobacter baumanii*, *Enterococcus* and *Candida* species identified in blood cultures. Tailored antibacterial and antifungal therapy including, daptomycin, caspofungin, meropenem, ceftazidim, linezolid, voriconazol, vancomycin, tigecyclin and anidulafungin was employed over 5 weeks. The patient was intubated and ventilated for 8 days. Acute renal failure required dialysis for 3 days. While the systemic infection markedly improved mucocutaneous lesions persisted. Consequently, topical clobetasol 0.05 % ointment (up to 300 g/day) and oral prednisolone (2 mg/kg) were initiated and after 1 week increased to 2.25 mg/kg. Two additional cycles of immunoadsorption and IVIG were given at 3 week intervals (Fig. 5.2). After 5 weeks the patient was discharged from ICU to the dermatology ward and mucocutaneous lesions started to improve allowing the cessation of treatment with topical corticosteroids steroids and tapering of the oral prednisolone dose. IVIG was further administered on a monthly basis while mycophenolate mofetil had to be reduced and later omitted due to increasing pancytopenia that was finally attributed to cytomegalovirus reactivation. Systemic antiviral therapy with valganciclovir for 8 weeks led to disappearance of the virus load. Ongoing bacteremia and systemic *Candida* infections required repeated systemic antimicrobial and antifungal therapy. Severe hyperkalaemia due to adrenal gland suppression was managed on ICU for few days. Since mucocutaneous lesions only healed slowly rituximab 1 g was given. However, the patient could be mobilized following intensive physiotherapy and was discharged to a rehabilitation hospital after nearly 6 months in our clinic with hydrocortisone 30 mg/day. He still had erosions on the back, upper arms, shoulders, nates and thighs covering about 1–2 % of his body surface corresponding to a PDAI of 18 (Fig. 5.3). Anti-desmoglein autoantibody levels had decreased by 97 % compared to admission (Fig. 5.2).

IVIG cycles were continued together with i.v. dexamethasone pulses (100 mg/day for three consecutive days) 4- and subsequently, 5-weekly. At present, 11 months after the first presentation in our department, the patient has a small post-traumatic erosion on his right upper arm while mucosal lesions had disappeared (Fig. 5.4). Anti-desmoglein 3 autoantibody levels are 71 U/ml with no anti-desmoglein 1 serum reactivity detectable (Fig. 5.2).

What was the single most important factor leading to recovery of this severely affected pemphigus vulgaris patient?

1. Dermatologists experienced in the treatment of severe pemphigus
2. Up-to date equipment of the ICU
3. Interdisciplinary team of motivated dermatologists, infectiologists, microbiologists, pharmacologists, nephrologists, anaesthesiologists, nurses, and physiotherapists
4. Regular monitoring of anti-desmoglein serum levels
5. High-dose corticosteroids

Discussion

Pemphigus vulgaris is a potentially life-threatening mucocutaneous autoimmune disorder [3]. Prior to the advent of systemic corticosteroids, the mortality associated with pemphigus vulgaris was up to 80 %. Today, a significant part of the associated mortality could be considered iatrogenic, i.e. related to side-effects of immunosuppressive therapy as illustrated by

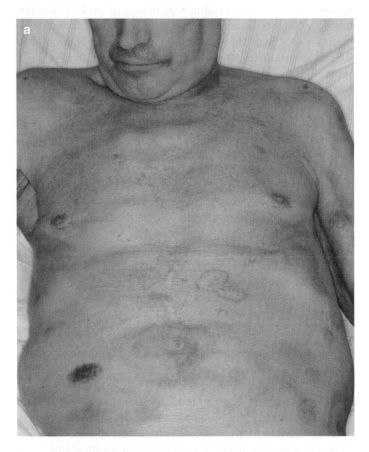

FIGURE 5.3 Small erosions on the chest, upper arms (**a**), shoulders, back (**b**), and nates, covering about 1–2 % of his body surface 6 months after the first presentation in our department

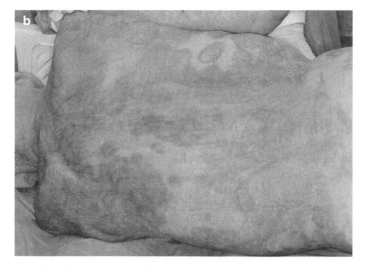

Figure 5.3 (continued)

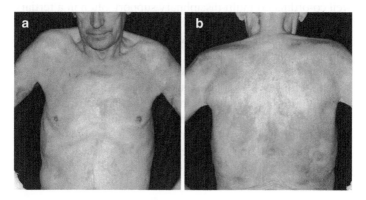

Figure 5.4 Small post-traumatic erosion on his right upper arm (a) 11 months after the first presentation in our clinic. On all other body sites (a, b) inclduing the oral mucosa, all lesions have healed

our case vignette. Pemphigus vulgaris most commonly develops during the fifth to seventh decades of life. Cutaneous lesions present as blisters and erosions on normal or erythematous skin. The oral mucosa is the initial site of involvement in the majority of cases and the clinical manifestations may indeed remain confined to the mucosal surfaces. However, in other cases skin changes may become more generalized. Diagnosis is based on the clinical manifestations combined with characteristic histological changes seen in lesional skin or mucosal biopsies, direct immunofluorescence microscopy of a perilesional biopsy, and the detection of serum anti-desmoglein 3 autoantibodies [4].

Therapeutic strategies rely on the use of systemic corticosteroids (prednisolone 1–2 mg/kg/day or i.v. dexamethasone pulses) in conjunction with other immunosuppressant agents such as azathioprine, mycophenolate mofetil or cyclophosphamide [5]. Rituximab (monoclonal anti-CD20 antibody), immunoadsorption und IVIG can be used in the treatment of refractory pemphigus vulgaris [6–9].

The presented case demonstrates that pemphigus vulgaris remains a potentially life-threatening disease. Treatment is limited by the range of serious side-effects associated with the current immunosuppressive therapy. Moreover, patients require well co-ordinated multi-disciplinary support, often in a tertiary referral center that has extensive expertise in the diagnosis and management of such a rare disease. Only the constant interaction between dermatologists, infectiologists, microbiologists, pharmacologists, nephrologists, anaesthiologists, nurses, and physiotherapists has enabled us to successfully manage this severely affected patient. Ultimately, the lack of randomized controlled trials in the management of pemphigus vulgaris [10] means that the choice of therapeutic regimen depends on several factors, including the patient's general medical condition, disease activity, treatment history and side-effect profile.

Key Points

- Pemphigus vulgaris is a potentially fatal autoimmune blistering disease characterized by erosions of mucous membranes and/or erosions and blisters of the skin.
- In pemphigus vulgaris, antibodies are directed against structural proteins of the epidermal desmosome, desmoglein 3, and in patients with skin involvement also desmoglein 1.

- Systemic corticosteroids are the therapeutic backbone of pemphigus vulgaris usually combined with additional immunosuppressants. In refractory cases, immunoadsorption, rituximab, and IVIG have successfully been applied.

References

1. Rosenbach M, Murrell DF, Bystryn JC, Dulay S, Dick S, Fakharzadeh S, Hall R, Korman NJ, Lin J, Okawa J, et al. Reliability and convergent validity of two outcome instruments for pemphigus. J Invest Dermatol. 2009;129:2404–10.
2. Zimmermann J, Bahmer F, Rose C, Zillikens D, Schmidt E. Clinical and immunopathological spectrum of paraneoplastic pemphigus. J Dtsch Dermatol Ges. 2010;8:598–605.
3. Stanley JR, Amagai M. Pemphigus, bullous impetigo, and the staphylococcal scalded-skin syndrome. N Engl J Med. 2006;355:1800–10.
4. Schmidt E, Zillikens D. Modern diagnosis of autoimmune blistering skin diseases. Autoimmun Rev. 2010;10:84–9.
5. Kasperkiewicz M, Schmidt E, Zillikens D. Current therapy of the pemphigus group. Clin Dermatol. 2012;30:84–94.
6. Ahmed AR, Spigelman Z, Cavacini LA, Posner MR. Treatment of pemphigus vulgaris with rituximab and intravenous immune globulin. N Engl J Med. 2006;355:1772–9.
7. Ishii N, Hashimoto T, Zillikens D, Ludwig RJ. High-dose intravenous immunoglobulin (IVIG) therapy in autoimmune skin blistering diseases. Clin Rev Allergy Immunol. 2010;38: 186–95.
8. Joly P, Mouquet H, Roujeau JC, D'Incan M, Gilbert D, Jacquot S, Gougeon ML, Bedane C, Muller R, Dreno B, et al. A single cycle of rituximab for the treatment of severe pemphigus. N Engl J Med. 2007;357:545–52.
9. Kasperkiewicz M, Shimanovich I, Meier M, Schumacher N, Westermann L, Kramer J, Zillikens D, Schmidt E. Treatment of severe pemphigus with a combination of immunoadsorption, rituximab, pulsed dexamethasone and azathioprine/mycophenolate mofetil: a pilot study of 23 patients. Br J Dermatol. 2012;166:154–60.
10. Martin LK, Werth V, Villanueva E, Segall J, Murrell DF. Interventions for pemphigus vulgaris and pemphigus foliaceus. Cochrane Database Syst Rev. 2009;1:CD006263.

Chapter 6
A Crusted Plaque on the Right Cheek in a 45 Year Old Woman

Maryam Ghiasi and Cheyda Chams-Davatchi

A 45-year-old woman presented with a 6×4 cm crusted plaque surrounded by erythema on her right cheek with the involvement of lower eyelid since 1 month ago (Fig. 6.1). She had a history of generalized blisters and erosions especially on the face, scalp and upper trunk and painful erosions on the lip and oral mucosa from a few years ago that was treated with systemic corticosteroids.

M. Ghiasi, M.D. (✉)
Autoimmune Bullous Diseases Research Center,
Department of Dermatology,
Tehran University of Medical Sciences,
Tehran, Iran

Autoimmune Bullous Diseases Research Center,
Razi Hospital, Vahdat Eslami Square,
Tehran, Iran
e-mail: mghiasi@tums.ac.ir

C. Chams-Davatchi, M.D.
Autoimmune Bullous Diseases Research Center,
Department of Dermatology,
Tehran University of Medical Sciences,
Tehran, Iran
e-mail: cchamsdavatchi@gmail.com

D.F. Murrell (ed.), *Clinical Cases in Autoimmune Blistering Diseases*, Clinical Cases in Dermatology 5, DOI 10.1007/978-3-319-10148-4_6, © Springer International Publishing Switzerland 2015

45

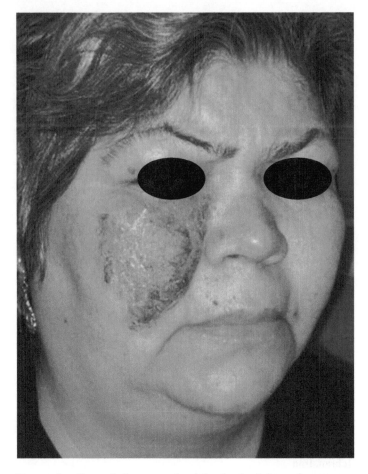

FIGURE 6.1 Crusted plaque on the right cheek of the patient

Based on the case description and photograph, what is your diagnosis?

1. Localized pemphigus vulgaris
2. Localized cicatricial pemphigoid
3. Impetigo
4. Dermatophytosis

Microscopic examination of the skin biopsy specimen revealed intraepidermal acantholysis supporting the diagnosis of pemphigus vulgaris (PV). Direct immunofluorescence showed intercellular staining with IgG and C3 in the epidermis.

Diagnosis

Localized Pemphigus Vulgaris

The first presentation of PV in this patient was multiple blisters and erosions on the face, scalp and upper trunk and erosions on the lip and oral mucosa. At that time, the patient was treated with systemic prednisolone and azathioprine. She had good response and prednisolone was tapered. Generalized PV recurred several times on low dose prednisolone. Recurrences were treated with increase in the dose of prednisolone. After a few years, a 6×4 cm crusted plaque surrounded by erythema appeared on her right cheek with the involvement of lower eyelid. Intralesional triamcinolone was injected several times with the diagnosis of localized PV. The lesion had partial improvement but recurred at the same site a couple of times.

Discussion

PV is an autoimmune blistering disease with autoantibodies against the cell surface of keratinocyte. Initial involvement of oral mucosa is a well-known feature of the disease seen in 50–70 % of patients. These lesions are usually followed by the onset of more disseminated ones, on the mucosa or on the skin, after a time lapse ranging from weeks to months [1].

Localized lesions of pemphigus can be the presenting feature of pemphigus. In the course of pemphigus, the lesions may remain localized before spreading over the whole integument but it is exceptional that the condition remains localized over 5 months [2]. However, pemphigus has been reported to remain localized for 7 years. Also, localized lesions of pemphigus can be the sole manifestation of pemphigus vulgaris.

Another form of localized PV can be established in the course of the disease after disseminated lesions had been subsided, as in our patient. This form of localized PV is not rare and in our experience it is not unusual that PV patients have some recurrent localized lesions after improvement of disseminated lesions.

The pathophysiology of localized pemphigus is not clearly established. Some cases of localized pemphigus that have been developed at sites of trauma, burns and surgical scars have been reported in the literature suggesting a koebner-like phenomenon [2]. Most cases of localized pemphigus occur on the face and scalp. This finding is consistent with the distribution of PV antigen which is strongly expressed in face, neck and scalp [3]. Also some theorize that localized pemphigus of the face and scalp may be triggered by ultraviolet radiation. This hypothesis is based on the experimental induction of acantholysis in pemphigus patients and clinical exacerbation of the diseases after sun exposure [4].

Intralesional steroid injection is a good therapeutic option for localized lesions of pemphigus. But it may be complicated by infection at injection sites, especially when the patient is immunocompromised as a result of systemic steroid and immunosuppressive agents, so aseptic technique should be used for intralesional injection in such patients.

Key Points

- Localized pemphigus is a variant of pemphigus that can be presented as the sole manifestation of pemphigus or in the course of the disease before or after disseminated lesions.
- The most common sites of localized PV are face and scalp.
- Intralesional steroid injection is the best treatment for localized PV.

References

1. Lapiere K, Caers S, Lambert J. A case of long-lasting localized pemphigus vulgaris of scalp. Dermatology. 2004;209(2):162–3.
2. Zaraa I, El Euch D, Kort R, et al. Localized pemphigus: a report of three cases. Int J Dermatol. 2010;49(6):715–6.
3. SisonFonacier BL, Bystryn JC. Regional variations in antigenic properties of skin. A possible cause for disease specific distributions of skin lesions. J Exp Med. 1986;164(6):2125–30.
4. Lehrhoff S, Miller K, Fischer M, et al. Localized pemphigus with vegetative features. Dermatol Online J. 2012;18(12):11.

Chapter 7
A 52 Year Old Man with Cerebriform Vegetating Masses on the Scalp

Maryam Daneshpazhooh and Cheyda Chams-Davatchi

In November 2013, a 52 year old man presented with two large nodular cerebriform vegetating masses in the temporal regions of the scalp extending to the occipital regions. These lesions had appeared and worsened during the preceding years. They resembled the folded pattern of cutis verticis gyrata and were studded with pustules in the follicular ostia. Hair was sparse to absent on the gyri and tufted folliculitis-like pattern was seen wherever clusters of hair emerged from sulci between folds

M. Daneshpazhooh, M.D. (✉)
Autoimmune Bullous Diseases Research Center,
Department of Dermatology,
Tehran University of Medical Sciences,
Tehran, Iran
e-mail: daneshpj@tums.ac.ir

C. Chams-Davatchi, M.D.
Autoimmune Bullous Diseases Research Center,
Department of Dermatology,
Tehran University of Medical Sciences,
Tehran, Iran
e-mail: cchamsdavatchi@gmail.com

D.F. Murrell (ed.), *Clinical Cases in Autoimmune Blistering Diseases*, Clinical Cases in Dermatology 5, DOI 10.1007/978-3-319-10148-4_7,
© Springer International Publishing Switzerland 2015

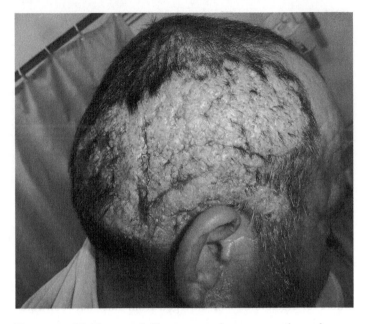

FIGURE 7.1 Hairless cerebriform vegetating mass on the scalp covered with pustules

(Fig. 7.1). Lesions were foul-smelling. The uninvolved occipital area showed mild skin folding of cutis verticis gyrata. Discrete erosions were also seen in the oral mucosa, as well as a few blisters on his trunk and left knee. He was receiving prednisolone 20 mg/day and methotrexate 10 mg/week. A deep biopsy was performed from his scalp. Suprabasal clefts, acantholysis and tombstone pattern were seen histopathologically. In addition, verrucous acanthosis, papillomatosis, epidermal hyperplasia and heavy dermal inflammatory infiltrate were prominent. Direct immunofluorescence was positive for intercellular epidermal IgG and C3 deposits. KOH smear was negative for fungi. In a culture from the scalp pustules *Staphylococcus aureus* was retrieved.

Based on the case description and the photograph, what is your diagnosis?

1. Pemphigus vegetans
2. Pemphigoid vegetans
3. Pyodermatitis-pyostomatitis vegetans
4. Wart

Diagnosis

Pemphigus Vegetans

In 2004 the patient presented with oral and skin bullae and erosions of 3 months duration. Oral biopsy and direct immunofluorescence were performed which showed suprabasal acantholysis and intercellular IgG and C3 deposits, respectively and were compatible with pemphigus vulgaris (PV). Treatment was started with prednisolone 1.5 mg/kg/day (120 mg/day) and azathioprine 2 g/kg (150 mg/day). After control of his condition, prednisolone was tapered gradually. He was unable to taper his prednisolone below 15 mg/day but was in complete control of his blistering at this dose, until 1 year later, when he experienced a minor relapse on the scalp, chest and oral mucosa when he was receiving prednisolone 15 mg/day and azathioprine 150 mg/day.

In the following years he never became free of scalp lesions. Only erosions and crusted lesions were seen initially. Lesions gradually showed features of tufted folliculitis, then progressed indolently to vegetating plaques. Pull test from the involved areas revealed anagen hair loss in the active phases of disease. The patient also experienced a few minor relapses involving the oral mucosa and skin besides his persistent progressive scalp lesions. Enzyme-linked immunosorbent assays were positive for anti-Dsg 3 (>200 U/ml) and negative for anti-Dsg 1 (<20 U/ml) on two occasions.

Adding Cellcept 2 g/day for 9 months, methotrexate 15 mg/ week for 5 months or minocycline 100 mg/day for a few months to the 15–30 mg prednisolone did not change the progressive course of his disease. Scalp lesions neither showed any response to multiple weekly intralesional injections of triamcinolone acetonide. The patient was never off treatment from steroids. He had poor compliance to treatments with irregular follow-up visits and suffered from uncontrolled diabetes mellitus.

His condition showed only some improvement while taking prednisolone 20 mg/day, methotrexate 20 mg/day as well as a course of clindamycin and ciprofloxacin, in his last visit in January 2014.

Figure 7.2 shows the dermoscopic view of the scalp examined in his last visit.

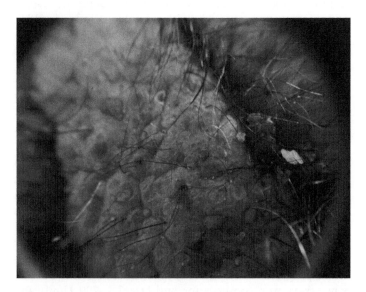

FIGURE 7.2 Dermoscopy of the scalp lesion showing vegetations, sparse hair, pustules and crusts in the empty follicular ostia

Discussion

PV is a chronic autoimmune blistering disease of the skin and/ or mucosa characterized by the presence of autoantibodies targeting desmoglein 3 and to a lesser extent desmoglein 1. Pemphigus vegetans (P Veg) is a rare clinical variant of PV and historically divided into Neumann and Hallopeau types, depending on the types of primary lesions and the clinical course. P Veg of Neumann type presents initially as PV with flaccid blisters and erosions. Its course is also similar to classical PV, however the erosions does evolve into vegetating verrucous excrescences especially in the intertriginous areas (axillae, groin, lip commisures). Local moisture, heat, friction, as well as secondary bacterial (*Staphylococcus aureus*) and fungal (*Candida albicans*) infections are important in the development and persistence of lesions. Management of vegetations is based on local hygiene, frequent bathing, local antiseptics and astringents, topical antibiotics, topical antifungals, oral antibiotics, and weekly intralesional triamcinolone injections. According to our experience, intralesional triamcinolone injections are usually effective. The dose of oral steroids should not be increased.

P Veg of Hallopeau type is very rare. It begins as pustules that gradually evolve into moist vegetating plaques. This type closely resembles pyodermatitis vegetans clinically. Patients with the Hallopeau type have a relatively benign course, require lower doses of systemic steroids, and usually have a prolonged remission.

Histopathologically, early lesions of P Veg show suprabasal acantholysis; however in established vegetating lesions epidermal hyperplasia, acanthosis and papillomatosis are seen. Intraepidermal microabscesses rich in eosinophils are conspicuous in the early stages of Hallopeau subtype. Immunofluorescence studies reveal intercellular epidermal IgG and/or C3 deposits. While antibodies against desmoglein 3 are consistently present in P Veg, anti-desmoglein 1 are only occasionally reported [1–4].

Pyodermatitis-pyostomatitis vegetans is a rare eosinophilic inflammatory dermatosis of unknown cause characterized by vesicular and pustular lesions and vegetating plaques. Oral cavity, skin folds and scalp are especially affected. It resembles P Veg both clinically and histologically; positive immunofluorescence findings seen in P Veg help differentiating these two diseases. Pyodermatitis-pyostomatitis vegetans is frequently associated with inflammatory bowel disease [5].

Pemphigoid gestationis is a very rare variant of bullous pemphigoid easily diagnosed by the presence of subepidermal blisters, Ig G and/or C3 deposit at the basement membrane zone and anti-BP 180 and 230 ELISA.

Extensive cutaneous warts may be a complication seen in immunosuppressed patients including patients with immunobullous diseases. Human papillomavirus infection can be ruled out by the absence of typical koilocytes in histopathological specimens.

Our patient had presented initially as a classical case of PV; however the progressive appearance of vegetating lesions on his scalp led us to the diagnosis of P Veg. Some aspects of this case are interesting and worth discussing:

1. The clinical appearance of the vegetating friable lesions was reminiscent to Hallopeau type, while the initial presentation and the course of the disease were similar to Neumann type. We have speculated that a classical PV may have been transformed into a localized P Veg of Hallopeau type over time; however pathological examination was not conclusive.

2. Intertriginous areas are usually affected in P Veg and isolated scalp involvement seen in this patient is rarely reported [4]. The grotesque cerebriform appearance of scalp lesions was also exceptional.

3. P Veg lesions in intertriginous areas usually respond to treatment; this was not the case for the scalp lesions in this patient which were intractable with a progressive course despite years of treatment. P Veg on the scalp appeared to be resistant to treatment according to a few previous case reports [4, 6]. Depending on the health system and funding, rituximab might be a good option for such a patient; it was

effective in resistant cases reported by Kim et al. and Kamphausen et al. [7, 8].

4. The lesions evolved through various stages of erosions, crusts, tufted folliculitis, anagen hair loss and exuberant vegetating overgrowth – various features of pemphigus seen in the scalp.

Key Pearls

P Veg should be considered in any patient with vegetating lesions in the body folds and scalp.

Scalp lesions in P Veg may be resistant to treatment.

Pyodermatitis-pyostomatitis is the most important differential of P Veg; direct immunofluorescence is helpful for confirming P Veg.

References

1. Zaraa I, Sellami A, Bouguerra C, Sellami MK, Chelly I, Zitouna M, Makni S, Hmida AB, Mokni M, Osman AB. Pemphigus vegetans: a clinical, histological, immunopathological and prognostic study. J Eur Acad Dermatol Venereol. 2011;25(10):1160–7.
2. Ahmed AR, Blose DA. Pemphigus vegetans. Neumann type and Hallopeau type. Int J Dermatol. 1984;23(2):135–41.
3. Cozzani E, Christana K, Mastrogiacomo A, Rampini P, Drosera M, Casu M, Murialdo G, Parodi A. Pemphigus vegetans Neumann type with anti-desmoglein and anti-periplakin autoantibodies. Eur J Dermatol. 2007;17(6):530–3.
4. Danopoulou I, Stavropoulos P, Stratigos A, Chatziolou E, Chiou A, Georgala S, Katsambas A. Pemphigus vegetans confined to the scalp. Int J Dermatol. 2006;45(8):1008–9.
5. Kitayama A, Misago N, Okawa T, Iwakiri R, Narisawa Y. Pyodermatitis-pyostomatitis vegetans after subtotal colectomy for ulcerative colitis. J Dermatol. 2010;37(8):714–7. Erratum in: J Dermatol. 2010 Sep;37(9):860.
6. Rackett SC, Rothe MJ, Hoss DM, Grin-Jorgensen CM, Grant-Kels JM. Treatment-resistant pemphigus vegetans of the scalp. Int J Dermatol. 1995;34(12):865–6.

7. Kim J, Teye K, Koga H, Yeoh SC, Wakefield D, Hashimoto T, Murrell DF. Successful single-cycle rituximab treatment in a patient with pemphigus vulgaris and squamous cell carcinoma of the tongue and IgG antibodies to desmocollins. J Am Acad Dermatol. 2013;69(1):e26–7.
8. Kamphausen I, Schulze F, Schmidt E, Zillikens D, Kunz M. Treatment of severe pemphigus vulgaris of the scalp with adjuvant rituximab and immunoadsorption. Eur J Dermatol. 2012;22(6): 786–7.

Chapter 8
Bullous Lesions on a Chronic Cutaneous Plaque

Vahide Lajevardi, Cheyda Chams-Davatchi,
Kamran Balighi, Ziba Rahbar, and Zahra Safaei-Naraghi

In March 2011, a 51-year-old man was referred to our department for his generalized mucocutaneous lesions. The onset of lesions was after an episode of a common cold 3 months earlier. He had an asymptomatic, erythematous plaque on the upper chest since childhood, and after his recent cold, the plaque became irritated, tender and multiple erosions

V. Lajevardi, M.D. (✉) • C. Chams-Davatchi, M.D.
Z. Rahbar, M.D.
Department of Dermatology,
Autoimmune Bullous Diseases Research Center,
Tehran University of Medical Sciences,
Tehran, Iran
e-mail: cchamsdavatchi@gmail.com; vahide_lajevardi@yahoo.com

K. Balighi, M.D.
Department of Dermatology, Autoimmune Bullous Research
Centre, Razi Hospital, Tehran University of Medical Sciences,
Vahdat Eslami, Tehran, Iran
e-mail: Kamran.balighi@yahoo.com

Z. Safaei-Naraghi, M.D.
Department of Dermatopathology, Autoimmune Bullous Research
Centre, Razi Hospital, Tehran University of Medical Sciences,
Vahdat Eslami, Tehran, Iran
e-mail: Zahra_s_naraghi@yahoo.com

D.F. Murrell (ed.), *Clinical Cases in Autoimmune*
Blistering Diseases, Clinical Cases in Dermatology 5,
DOI 10.1007/978-3-319-10148-4_8,
© Springer International Publishing Switzerland 2015

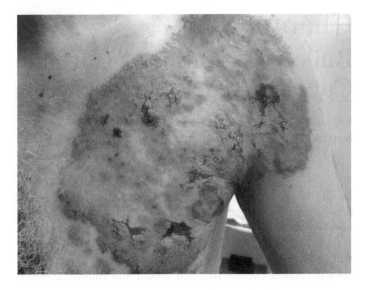

Figure 8.1 Multiple erosions and loose blisters on the base of the red brown indurated plaque with raised sharp borders and atrophic center on right upper chest with extension to the arm

and crusts appeared on it. Later the satellite lesions spread beyond the edge and 2 weeks before the referral, the eruptions became generalized. He had no history of similar lesions. Clinical examination revealed multiple erosions and loose blisters mostly on the left upper chest, erythematous plaque and scattered erosions on the scalp, face, trunk, limbs and oral mucosa (Fig. 8.1a). Sensation on the chest plaque appeared normal. The results of all laboratory tests were within normal ranges, except purified protein derivative (PPD)-tuberculin skin test that was positive with a 15 mm of induration. Histologic examination of a skin biopsy from the erosions on the old erythematous plaque of the chest, revealed focal supra-basal acantholysis within the epidermis, with bullae formation, while dense granulomatous aggregations of tuberculoid and foreign body type granulomas were seen in the upper and mid dermis. Areas of effacement of dermo-epidermal junction (DEJ) and interface pattern were also noted (Fig. 8.2).

Based on the case description and photograph, what is your diagnosis?

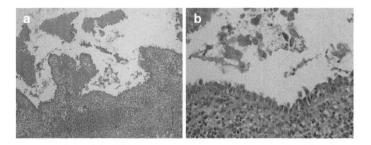

FIGURE 8.2 (**a**) Suprabasilar acantholysis within the epidermis. Dense granulomatous aggregations in the dermis. (**b**) row of tombstones appearance of the basal cells

1. Pemphigus vulgaris developed on cutaneous tuberculosis
2. Transient acantholytic dermatosis
3. bullous sarcoidosis
4. bullous lupus erythematosus

Diagnosis

Pemphigus vulgaris on a background of cutaneous tuberculosis (Lupus Vulgaris)

PCR evaluation for Mycobacterium tuberculosis (TB) DNA within the tissue was positive. Direct Immuno Fluorescence (DIF) examination revealed the intercellular IgG and C3 deposition.

The patient was treated with Isoniazid (300 mg/day), Pyrazinamide (1,750 mg/day), Ethambutol (1 g/day) mg/day and Prednisolone 100 mg/day. The lesions were significantly improved in 2 months (Fig. 8.1b). The anti-TB regimen was completed for 6 months and the steroid was tapered (Fig. 8.3). He was on complete remission on therapy in the 1 year follow up.

Discussion

Our patient presented for the first time in the literature the PV induced on the site of cutaneous tuberculosis. The diagnoses were confirmed through histopathology, PCR and DIF

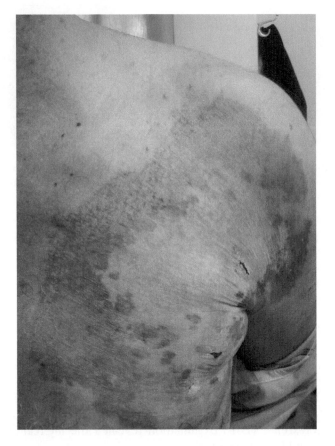

FIGURE 8.3 Improvement of lesions in 6 moth follow up shows the post inflammatory hyperpigmentation and central scar

evaluations and the lesions responded to the treatment of oral corticosteroid for PV and three-drug regimen for Lupus Vulgaris.

There are avfaew cases demonstrating the initial localization of pemphigus on the site of pre-existing dermatosese [1] and cutaneous injuries such as surgery [2], radiation [3, 4], cosmetic procedure [5] and burns [6]. Meanwhile, more than a chance finding, these would be potential interests for further research on the pathogenesis. It is also unusual for lupus vulgaris to only present on the chest without facial involvement and without a vaccination.

Lupus Vulgaris implies a strongly positive delayed hypersensitivity reaction to tuberculin with variable but prominent granulomata with little caseation in superficial dermis and bacteria are infrequent. It is contracted either by inoculation or by hematogenous dissemination and as the plaque expands the scarring develops centrally [7]. To answer the question of how these two rare diseases were linked, a complex interaction of genetic, local, and systemic factors that influence the immune responses is probably responsible. One interesting possibility would be the decreased expression of Interleukin 12 receptor that has been detected in pemphigus [8] and its heritable deficiency was also linked to susceptibility to tuberculosis [9], however that was not evaluated for our patient. Injuries that disturb the DEJ in traumatized epithelium, could further express epidermal antigens, expose new epitopes or enhance antigen presenting to initiate antibody formation in genetically predisposed patients [10, 11], and it was noted it our specimens. Also, chronic stimulation of the immune system in that site, coupled with epithelial damage in a susceptible individual. Also, altered target antigens presented by infected cell and deposits of circulating immune complexes in the traumatized area could predispose to trigger the onset of an autoimmune blistering skin.

Key Points

Skin injuries such as surgical scar, burning and radiation that disturb the DEJ in traumatized epithelium, could express epidermal antigens, expose new epitopes or enhance antigen presenting to initiate antibody formation in genetically predisposed. They can be considered to be local factors which facilitate the autoimmune response of pemphigus, which in turn may induce blistering cutaneous lesions in subclinical patients with autoantibodies.

References

1. Lee CW, Ro YS. Pemphigus developed on preexisting dermatoses. J Dermatol. 1994;21(3):213–5.
2. Reichert-Penetrat S, Barbaud A, Martin S, Omhover L, Weber M, Schmutz JL. Pemphigus vulgaris on an old surgical scar: Koebner's phenomenon? Eur J Dermatol EJD. 1998;8(1):60–2.
3. Ambay A, Stratman E. Ionizing radiation-induced pemphigus foliaceus. J Am Acad Dermatol. 2006;54(5 Suppl):251–2.
4. Kim J, Teye K, Koga H, Yeoh S-C, Wakefield D, Hashimoto T, et al. Successful single-cycle rituximab treatment in a patient with pemphigus vulgaris and squamous cell carcinoma of the tongue and IgG antibodies to desmocollins. J Am Acad Dermatol. 2013 Jul;69(1):e26–27.
5. Kaplan RP, Detwiler SP, Saperstein HW. Physically induced pemphigus after cosmetic procedures. Int J Dermatol. 1993;32(2):100–3.
6. Hogan P. Pemphigus vulgaris following a cutaneous thermal burn. Int J Dermatol. 1992;31(1):46–9.
7. Sehgal VN, Sehgal R, Bajaj P, Sriviastava G, Bhattacharya S. Tuberculosis verrucosa cutis (TBVC). J Eur Acad Dermatol Venereol JEADV. 2000;14(4):319–21.
8. Takahashi H, Amagai M, Tanikawa A, et al. T helper type 2-biased natural killer cell phenotype in patients with pemphigus vulgaris. J Invest Dermatol. 2007;127(2):324–30.
9. De Beaucoudrey L, Samarina A, Bustamante J, et al. Revisiting human IL-12Rβ1 deficiency: a survey of 141 patients from 30 countries. Medicine (Baltimore). 2010;89(6):381–402.
10. Rotunda AM, Bhupathy AR, Dye R, Soriano TT. Pemphigus foliaceus masquerading as postoperative wound infection: report of a case and review of the Koebner and related phenomenon following surgical procedures. Dermatol Surg. 2006;31(2):226–31.
11. Pérez-Pérez L, Suárez O, Sánchez-Aguilar D, Toribio J. Pemphigus vulgaris beginning as the Koebner phenomenon. Actas Dermosifiliogr. 2005;96(10):681–4.

Chapter 9
A 60-Year-Old Woman with Pemphigus Vulgaris Refractory to High-Dose Prednisone

Elizabeth S. Robinson and Victoria P. Werth

A 60-year-old woman weighing 55 kg presented to the clinic with a 4-month history of sores in her mouth and on her chest. Skin biopsy showed a sparse, superficial, perivascular dermatitis with suprabasal acantholysis. Direct immunofluorescence was positive for IgG and C3 in an intercellular pattern. The patient was started on prednisone at 80 mg per day by an outside dermatologist 1 month prior to referral. Her disease flared when she attempted to taper the prednisone below 80 mg per day, with painful erosions that interfered with eating on her left and right buccal mucosa, and on the left side of her mouth, as well as extensive erosions on her chest and back, and some erosions on her legs.

Based on the case description, what is the next step in treatment?

E.S. Robinson, BSE • V.P. Werth, M.D. (✉)
Philadelphia Veteran Affairs Medical Center,
Philadelphia, PA USA

Department of Dermatology, University of Pennsylvania,
14 Penn Tower, Room 1430, 1 Convention Ave.,
Philadelphia, PA 19104, USA
e-mail: esr2133@columbia.edu; werth@mail.med.upenn.edu

D.F. Murrell (ed.), *Clinical Cases in Autoimmune Blistering Diseases*, Clinical Cases in Dermatology 5, DOI 10.1007/978-3-319-10148-4_9, © Springer International Publishing Switzerland 2015

Treatment

Adjuvant rituximab

Discussion

Pemphigus vulgaris (PV) is a potentially life-threatening autoimmune bullous dermatosis of the skin and/or mucous membranes caused by autoantibodies against the cadherins desmoglein 1 and desmoglein 3. Standard treatment of PV requires high-dose prednisone at 1–2 mg/kg/day that may be combined with other immunosuppressive medications such as cyclophosphamide, methotrexate, azathioprine, or mycophenolate mofetil. Per the International Pemphigus Committee's 2008 consensus statement, failure of PV therapy is defined as the, "continued development of new lesions, continued extension of old lesions, or failure of established lesions to begin to heal despite 3 weeks of therapy on 1.5 mg/kg/day of prednisone" with or without the additional immunosuppressive agents mentioned above [1].

For patients with refractory PV, contraindications to immunosuppressive therapies, and/or severe and debilitating PV that will not likely respond to a standard treatment regimen, therapy focuses on depleting the desmoglein antibodies. Rituximab and/or intravenous immunoglobulin (IVIG) are used in such cases. Rituximab is generally preferred due to the better side effect profile and lower cost.

Rituximab

Rituximab is an IgG antibody that targets the CD20 antigen of B lymphocytes, the precursor cell to antibody producing plasma cells. It depletes the pathogenic desmoglein antibodies in PV for 6–12 months [2]. Rituximab is FDA approved for various leukemias and lymphomas, rheumatoid arthritis, and some vasculitides. It is used off-label for PV.

The optimal dosing protocol of rituximab for PV treatment is unclear. Initial PV treatment with rituximab used the lymphoma dosing protocol of four weekly 375 mg/m^2 infusions. More recent studies examined the use of the rheumatoid arthritis dosing of 1,000 mg twice, 2 weeks apart. In a meta-analysis of 42 case reports and case series from 2000 to 2012 of rituximab therapy in PV patients recalcitrant to standard therapies, complete remission was achieved in 67 % (32/48) of patients from case reports and in 67 % (56/84) of patients from case series using the lymphoma protocol compared to 79 % (n = 59/75) of patients from case series following the RA protocol [3]. Both dosing protocols required the concurrent use of prednisone and/or other systemic therapies. Seven patients following the lymphoma protocol did not respond to treatment, while no patients on the RA protocol were non-responders. Relapse occurred in 23 % (30/132) of patients on the lymphoma protocol and in 36 % (27/75) on the RA protocol. Overall, this meta-analysis found that patients in the RA protocol had a higher response rate, a higher relapse rate, a higher number of infections, and a lower mortality rate compared to the lymphoma protocol. A recent, prospective, randomized, observer blinded study of 22 patients with PV or pemphigus foliaceus (PF) found no difference in time to disease control between patients treated with low dose rituximab (two 500 mg doses, 15 days apart) compared to the higher dose RA protocol, although relapse was more common and more adjuvant immunosuppressive therapy was needed in the low dose group [4].

A multicenter, prospective study of 14 PV patients with refractory disease treated with a single cycle of rituximab using the lymphoma protocol suggests that a second cycle of rituximab may be required only in relapse that cannot be controlled with first-line therapies. This study reported that 86 % (12/14) of subjects had complete remission of disease (defined as the epithelization of all skin and mucosal lesions) 3 months after the last infusion [5]. Of the remaining two subjects, one had complete remission by 180 days and the other by 360 days. All patients that were concurrently treated with steroids were able to significantly reduce their baseline prednisone dose. At the 34 month follow-up, 57 % (8/14) of subjects remained free of disease.

In a later study, Lunardon et al. found that 100 % (24/24) of severe and/or refractory PV patients treated with rituximab had clinical disease activity improvement [6]. Patients were treated with either the lymphoma or RA dosing protocol for up to four cycles if needed to improve the clinical outcome or to treat relapses. 58 % (14/24) of patients reached the study endpoint: complete remission on no or minimal systemic therapy. There was no significant difference between the two protocols in achieving this end point. In addition, 46 % of patients (11/24) attained complete remission on no systemic therapy. Of note, the study examined an additional seven patients with PF and found similar results. The median relapse-free remission time of the combined PV and PF patients was 19 months. This study also found a significant decrease in the serum desmoglein index value (median change of −80 %) in ten paired serum samples of patients before and after therapy. Finally, the study found that treatment with rituximab earlier in the disease course yielded better outcomes. The median duration of disease prior to rituximab therapy was 19 months for patients who achieved complete remission on no or minimal systemic therapy compared to 86 months for patients who did not. The mechanism of incomplete remission and/or relapse in some PV patients treated with rituximab is unclear, but may be attributed to persistent B cells in the spleen or lymph nodes, or new bone marrow-derived B cells with novel immunoglobulin rearrangements [7].

The most common side effects of rituximab treatment are mild, infusion-related events such as headache, fever, chills, nausea, pruritus, and hypotension that can be reduced with premedication. The most concerning adverse effect is serious and/or fatal infections [8, 9]. In a recent study of rituximab therapy in ANCA-associated vasculitides, severe infections occurred in 15 % (12/80) of patients and caused four deaths (5 %) [10]. Late-onset infections are possible, occurring up to 85 months after the first rituximab dose, and up to 10 months after the last rituximab dose in a study of 17 patients with vasculitis followed for at least 3 years [11]. It is unclear if the increased risk of infection is due to rituximab itself, secondary to a reduced number of B cells, or from the multiple immunosuppressive therapies that patients are often taking concurrently, particularly because some patients with normal IgG levels experienced serious infections [5]. Patients with severe infections should not receive rituximab. Patients should be tested for tuberculosis and hepatitis prior to rituximab therapy, as well as receive immunizations such as pneumovax, if age appropriate.

Screening for hepatitis B virus (HBV) must include tests for both the hepatitis B surface antigen (HBsAg) and the hepatitis B core antibody (anti-HBc) prior to the initiation of treatment. In September 2013, the FDA issued a new *Boxed Warning* for rituximab following 109 cases of fatal HBV induced acute liver injury, including cases of HBV reactivation in patients with previously resolved HBV infections (HBsAg-, anti-HBc+, and hepatitis B surface antibody [anti-HBs]+) [12]. Patients with prior HBV infection should be monitored for signs and symptoms of HBV reactivation both during and after the rituximab treatment by PCR for hepatitis B virus. If a patient experiences reactivation of HBV, an antiviral therapy should be initiated.

Other adverse events of rituximab therapy include: allergic infusion reactions, leukopenia, lymphopenia, neutropenia, and persistent hypogammaglobulinemia. Overall, rituximab is well tolerated and the side effects are moderate compared to the adverse effects of long-term, high-dose corticosteroids and other immunosuppressive agents. However, its use should be limited to severe, refractory PV because of the possible side effects.

IVIG

The exact mechanism of action of IVIG in the treatment of PV is unclear. IVIG may have immunomodulatory actions on both B and T cell function, reduce serum levels of anti-desmoglein antibodies, and/or modify the function of the Fc receptor [13, 14]. The first randomized, placebo-controlled, double-blind trial with IVIG in pemphigus was reported in 2009 [15]. Twenty-one patients with PV and PF received 400 mg/kg/day of IVIG; 20 patients received 200 mg/kg/day of IVIG; and, 20 patients received placebo. Each patient group received five consecutive days of treatment with the assigned therapy. The time to escape from the protocol (the time until additional treatment was needed) was significantly prolonged for the 400 mg/kg/day group compared to the placebo group ($P < 0.001$), and a dose-response relationship in this outcome was observed among the three groups. There was no significant difference in adverse drug reactions among the three arms.

While the use of IVIG in PV has a corticosteroid sparing effect, [16] IVIG should be used prudently due to its expense (often greater than $100,000 a year) and side effect profile. The most concerning adverse effect of IVIG is thrombotic events, such as stroke or myocardial infarction. No study has quantified the incidence of thrombotic events with IVIG therapy in PV. In the authors' experience, the high incidence of thrombosis is concerning and requires caution, especially as PV patients may have anticardiolipin antibodies that already predispose them to thrombotic events. Further studies on the incidence of thrombosis during IVIG therapy are needed.

The most common side effect of IVIG is an infusion-related headache. Such headaches can be reduced with a slower infusion rate and acetaminophen. Other adverse effects of IVIG include: chills, hypotension, fever, myalgias, nausea, vomiting, infusion-site reactions, hemolysis, neutropenia, anaphylaxis in IgA deficiency, aseptic meningitis, and the potential to transfuse infectious agents.

Rituximab and IVIG

IVIG may be added to rituximab therapy in PV to hasten disease resolution. IVIG may also provide protection from rituximab-induced hypogammaglobulinemia, and may therefore decrease the risk of infection with rituximab. However, infection with rituximab therapy may occur up to 18 months after treatment, [5] which would not be prevented by combined rituximab and IVIG treatment early in PV therapy.

A study of 11 patients with PV refractory to conventional therapy or IVIG that were treated with a combination of IVIG and rituximab found that nine patients had rapid resolution of their clinical pemphigus disease activity lasting 22–37 months [17]. All 11 patients were able to discontinue all additional immunosuppressive therapies before the end of the study. This study reported no clinically significant adverse effects, including no infections.

Key Points

- Rituximab is the mainstay of treatment for patients with severe PV that is refractory to standard treatments. It produces complete remission in over 65 % of patients, and enables patients to reduce or discontinue toxic immunosuppressive therapies. Rituximab is more effective if used early in the course of PV.
- IVIG may be used alone or in combination with rituximab to more quickly reduce disease activity, but should be reserved for patients with severe disease due to its high cost and risk of thrombotic events.

References

1. Murrell DF, Dick S, Ahmed AR, et al. Consensus statement on definitions of disease, end points, and therapeutic response for pemphigus. J Am Acad Dermatol. 2008;58(6):1043–6.
2. Browning JL. B cells move to centre stage: novel opportunities for autoimmune disease treatment. Nat Rev Drug Discov. 2006;5(7):564–76.
3. Zakka LR, Shetty SS, Ahmed AR. Rituximab in the treatment of pemphigus vulgaris. Dermatol Ther. 2012;2(1):17.
4. Kanwar AJ, Vinay K, Sawatkar GU, et al. Clinical and immunological outcomes of high- and low-dose rituximab treatments in

patients with pemphigus: a randomized, comparative, observer-blinded study. Br J Dermatol. 2014;170(6):1341–9.

5. Joly P, Mouquet H, Roujeau JC, et al. A single cycle of rituximab for the treatment of severe pemphigus. N Engl J Med. 2007;357(6):545–52.

6. Lunardon L, Tsai KJ, Propert KJ, et al. Adjuvant rituximab therapy of pemphigus: a single-center experience with 31 patients. Arch Dermatol. 2012;148(9):1031–6.

7. Leandro MJ, Cambridge G, Ehrenstein MR, Edwards JC. Reconstitution of peripheral blood B cells after depletion with rituximab in patients with rheumatoid arthritis. Arthritis Rheum. 2006;54(2):613–20.

8. Dupuy A, Viguier M, Bedane C, et al. Treatment of refractory pemphigus vulgaris with rituximab (anti-CD20 monoclonal antibody). Arch Dermatol. 2004;140(1):91–6.

9. Morrison LH. Therapy of refractory pemphigus vulgaris with monoclonal anti-CD20 antibody (rituximab). J Am Acad Dermatol. 2004;51(5):817–9.

10. Charles P, Neel A, Tieulie N, et al. Rituximab for induction and maintenance treatment of ANCA-associated vasculitides: a multicentre retrospective study on 80 patients. Rheumatology. 2014;53(3):532–9.

11. Pearce F, Lanyon P. Long-term efficacy and safety of rituximab in ANCA-associated vasculitis: results from a UK tertiary referral center. British Society for Rheumatology annual meeting 2014, Abstract 333.

12. Boxed Warning and new recommendations to decrease risk of hepatitis B reactivation with the immune-suppressing and anti-cancer drugs Arzerra (ofatumumab) and Rituxan (rituximab). 25 Sep 2013. http://www.fda.gov/downloads/Drugs/DrugSafety/UCM369436.pdf. Accessed 15 Apr 2014.

13. Kazatchkine MD, Kaveri SV. Immunomodulation of autoimmune and inflammatory diseases with intravenous immune globulin. N Engl J Med. 2001;345(10):747–55.

14. Li N, Zhao M, Hilario-Vargas J, et al. Complete FcRn dependence for intravenous Ig therapy in autoimmune skin blistering diseases. J Clin Invest. 2005;115(12):3440–50.

15. Amagai M, Ikeda S, Shimizu H, et al. A randomized double-blind trial of intravenous immunoglobulin for pemphigus. J Am Acad Dermatol. 2009;60(4):595–603.

16. Sami N, Qureshi A, Ruocco E, Ahmed AR. Corticosteroid-sparing effect of intravenous immunoglobulin therapy in patients with pemphigus vulgaris. Arch Dermatol. 2002;138(9):1158–62.
17. Ahmed AR, Spigelman Z, Cavacini LA, Posner MR. Treatment of pemphigus vulgaris with rituximab and intravenous immune globulin. N Engl J Med. 2006;355(17):1772–9.

Chapter 10
Beware of Infection: 48-Year Old Woman with Refractory Mucocutaneous Blisters

Julia S. Lehman

A 48-year-old previously healthy woman presented with 3 months of worsening weeping mucocutaneous erosions, generalized weakness, and malaise (Figure). A skin biopsy for routine microscopy and direct immunofluorescence confirmed the diagnosis. Despite treatment with systemic corticosteroids (oral and intramuscular) and topical corticosteroids, she continued to develop new lesions. She had not been taking any medications prior to the onset of the rash.

Based on the case description and the photograph (Fig. 10.1), what is your diagnosis?

(A) Bullous pemphigoid, with superinfection
(B) Pemphigus vulgaris, with superinfection
(C) Linear IgA bullous dermatosis, with superinfection
(D) Disseminated herpes zoster infection

The patient was hospitalized for multidisciplinary care. Routine microscopy showed suprabasilar acantholysis, and direct immunofluorescence showed cell-surface deposition of

J.S. Lehman, M.D., FAAD
Department of Dermatology and Laboratory Medicine and
Pathology, Mayo Clinic, Rochester, MN, USA
e-mail: Lehman.Julia@mayo.edu

D.F. Murrell (ed.), *Clinical Cases in Autoimmune*
Blistering Diseases, Clinical Cases in Dermatology 5,
DOI 10.1007/978-3-319-10148-4_10,
© Springer International Publishing Switzerland 2015

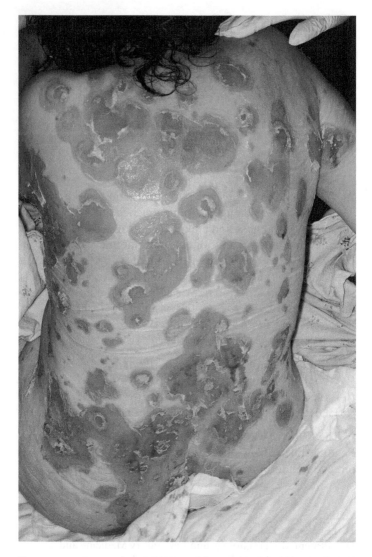

FIGURE 10.1 In a patient with pemphigus vulgaris, widespread cutaneous erosions with polymicrobial colonization

IgG and C3. Serum enzyme-linked immunosorbent assays for desmogleins 1 and 3 showed them to be markedly elevated (210 and 181 units, respectively). Skin swabs were positive for herpes simplex virus I by polymerase chain reaction and *Candida parapsilosis*, *Enterobacter*, methicillin-sensitive *Staphylococcus aureus*, and Pseudomonas aeruginosa by culture.

Diagnosis

Pemphigus Vulgaris, with Superinfection

Pemphigus vulgaris results when autoantibodies develop against keratinocyte adhesion molecules called desmogleins [1]. Affected patients experience painful oral erosions and often also develop fragile blisters and erosions of the skin. Therapy usually requires potent immunosuppressive medications, including high-dose corticosteroids, rituximab, or other steroid-sparing immunosuppressive agents [1].

The breach in the mucocutaneous barrier coupled with iatrogenic immunosuppression places affected patients at risk for superinfection of skin lesions [2–4]. Frequently implicated organisms include bacteria (especially *Staphylococcus aureus* and *E. coli*), viruses (especially herpes simplex virus and varicella zoster virus), and fungi (especially *Candida* sp.; [3]).

Given the severity of the patient's pemphigus vulgaris, tapering high-dose intravenous corticosteroids and mycophenolate mofetil were initiated on admission. To treat the patient's superinfection, systemic antimicrobial agents, potassium permanganate whirlpool baths, and antiseptic wet dressings with topical corticosteroids were also administered. After the first few weeks of therapy, she had experienced only modest improvement in her skin erosions despite skin cultures reverting to negative. Then, a serum mycophenolate acid trough level was checked and found to be subtherapeutic, despite appropriate dosing. Therefore, rituximab infusions weekly over 4 weeks were initiated in place of mycophenolate mofetil. Careful attention was paid to her nutritional and pain status throughout hospitalization. Her course was complicated by systemic inflammatory response syndrome and electrolyte imbalances requiring transfer to the intensive care unit, as well as opioid-associated delirium. Following a 2-month inpatient hospitalization, her mucocutaneous surface eventually completely re-epithelialized. She is doing well on azathioprine monotherapy after 1 year of clinical follow-up.

Key Points

- Patients with pemphigus vulgaris may develop superinfection by bacteria, viruses (especially herpes simplex virus and varicella zoster virus), and fungi (especially *Candida* sp.).
- In all patients with immunobullous diseases that are not responding to appropriate therapies, it is essential to consider the possibility of superinfection. Ideally, infections should be treated (and age-appropriate immunizations should be administered) prior to initiation or escalation of systemic immunosuppressive therapies.

References

1. Venugopal SS, Murrell DF. Diagnosis and clinical features of pemphigus vulgaris. Dermatol Clin. 2011;29(3):373–80.
2. Lehman JS, Murrell DF, Camilleri MJ, Kalaaji AN. Infection and infection prevention in patients treated with immunosuppressive medications for autoimmune bullous disorders. Dermatol Clin. 2011;29(4):591–8.
3. Esmaili N, Mortazavi H, Noormohammadpour P, Boreiri M, et al. Pemphigus vulgaris and infections: a retrospective study on 155 patients. Autoimmun Dis. 2013;2013:83295.
4. Lehman JS, Khunger M, Lohse CM. Infection in autoimmune bullous diseases: a retrospective comparative study. J Dermatol. 2013;40(8):613–9.

Chapter 11
A 71-Year-Old Man with Blisters on the Face and a Painful Left Thigh

Xinyi Yang, Melanie Joy C. Doria, and Dédée F. Murrell

A 71-year-old, Caucasian male being treated for pemphigus vulgaris (PV) by his local doctor with methotrexate 20 mg/week was referred with an 8-week history of grouped vesicles, some with erosions on the right side of the face (Fig. 11.1) and a 4-week history of a painful left anterolateral thigh. He had been diagnosed with PV 3 years previously and had been on prednisone for 19 months; the highest dose given was 100 mg/day. He had previously reacted badly to cyclophosphamide and azathioprine. His systemic steroid was gradually being tapered depending on his response to the medication. His last flare up was 3 months earlier, after which he was started on methotrexate 30 mg/week. Prior to this admission, he had achieved control of disease activity of his PV and was managed with prednisone 50 mg/day and methotrexate 20 mg/week.

On examination, he had grouped, red erythematous vesicles, some with erosions topped with crust on the right side of

X. Yang
University of New South Wales, Sydney, UNSW, Australia

M.J.C. Doria • D.F. Murrell, M.A., BMBCh, M.D., FAAD, FACD (✉)
University of New South Wales, Sydney, NSW, Australia

Department of Dermatology, St George Hospital,
Sydney, NSW, Australia
e-mail: d.murrell@unsw.edu.au

D.F. Murrell (ed.), *Clinical Cases in Autoimmune Blistering Diseases*, Clinical Cases in Dermatology 5, DOI 10.1007/978-3-319-10148-4_11,
© Springer International Publishing Switzerland 2015

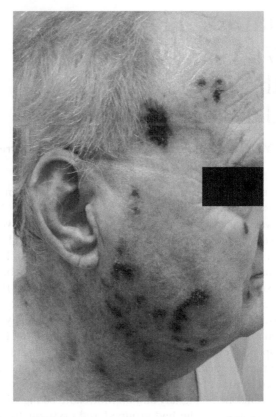

FIGURE 11.1 Ill defined, grouped, erythematous vesicles, some with erosions topped with crust on the right side of the face

the face (Fig. 11.1). Further examination showed well-defined, red erythematous patches and plaques with erosions on the posterior thighs; these lesions were noted few weeks before the onset of the painful left thigh (Fig. 11.2).

There was no fever, vomiting, headache, anorexia, weakness, cough or joint pain. No abnormality was detected on blood tests and X-ray of the left femur. Based on the case description and photograph, what are your diagnoses?

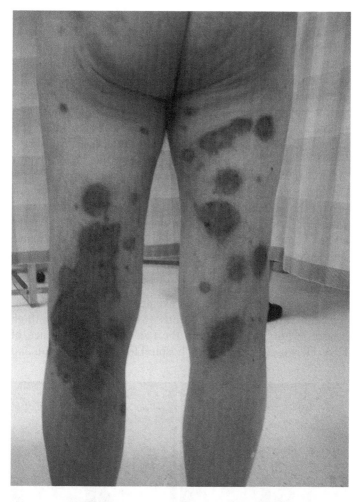

FIGURE 11.2 PV flare-up 7 weeks prior to the current admission (*left*)

1. PV (flare-up) and cellulitis
2. Herpes Zoster and abscess
3. Impetigo and cellulitis
4. Herpes simplex virus (HSV) infection and abscess

Core temperature was measured to detect constitutional signs for systemic infection despite the absence of fever, chills and sweats on patient history. Skin swab of the erosions on the face was sent for viral PCR testing, Gram stain and bacterial culture. Samples of the thigh swelling were taken for bacterial culture using ultrasound-guided percutaneous aspiration, but the residual amount of pus was significant, with reoccurrence of abscess. Follow-up CT scans showed loculated abscesses within the left adductor muscles (Fig. 11.3).

The largest collection was located in the left adductor magnus, measuring $3 \times 3 \times 7$ cm in antero-posterior, transverse and craniocaudal diameter. The small collection lied superiorly in the adductor brevis muscle, measuring 2.5 cm. There were poorly circumscribed, low-density changes in the right adductor brevis muscles, measuring 1.8 cm in the axial plane. This suggested the formation of an early collection at an adjacent site.

Empirical treatment of valaciclovir 500 mg bd for herpes was initiated. Bacterial culture revealed growth of Methicillin-Resistant Staphylococcus aureus (MRSA) from the thigh abscess, while the lesions on the face revealed presence of HSV. He was admitted to the hospital for further incision and

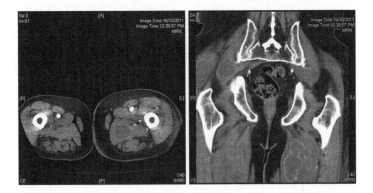

FIGURE 11.3 CT scan with contrast of the thighs showing bilateral collections within the adductor muscles; transverse section (*left*), coronal view (*right*)

drainage of the left thigh abscess in the operating theatre. He was given intravenous vancomycin therapy for 2 weeks. Upon completion of vancomycin, he was discharged with oral rifampicin 300 mg bd and fusidic acid 500 mg bd for 1 month to treat the MRSA infection. The valaciclovir was continued for the treatment of HSV infection. Methotrexate was discontinued, while prednisone was tapered to 40 mg/day from the week of admission until discharge. After the antibiotics regime, he was started on mycophenolate mofetil as adjuvant treatment for his PV.

Diagnosis

Herpes simplex virus (HSV) infection and abscess

Discussion

PV is an autoimmune intraepithelial blistering disease affecting mucosal and/or cutaneous tissues due to IgG antibodies attacking desmosomes leading to loss of cell-cell adhesion of keratinocytes, resulting in acantholysis [2]. Patients with autoimmune blistering conditions are susceptible to systemic infection due to long term use of immunosuppressive medications, which are the mainstay of treatment. The patients are also predisposed to developing secondary skin infections due to epidermal damage when vesicles rupture and release exudates that nurture pathogen colonisation. In addition, patients with autoimmune disease have deregulated innate immunity [14]. Higher infection risk is associated with multiple hospital admissions, increased disease severity and presence of diabetes mellitus. Staphylococcal aureus and Escherichia coli are common infective agents and 9.68–17 % of PV patients may suffer from localised herpes virus infection [8].

There have been multiple reports on the association of HSV infection and PV, especially in cases of relapse of PV or in patients who are unresponsive to immunosuppressive therapy [4, 5, 6]. HSV is transmitted through direct contact of infectious secretion with the mucous membrane or damaged skin. It may be latent in the ganglia, or reactivate as the virus travels through peripheral sensory nerves to the skin [3].

Immunosuppression is associated with higher frequencies of atypical HSV presentations, such as larger lesions, deeper ulceration, delayed wound healing and satellite lesions. HSV infection in immunocompromised hosts can mimic PV flare-up [6]. A negative Tzanck test cannot exclude the possibility of HSV infection; therefore PCR, electron microscopy and viral culture are better diagnostic tests to verify clinical diagnosis. Skin swab of new and intact blister is recommended over eroded or crusted lesions due to less contamination and higher sensitivity [9]. Indicated treatment options for HSV include oral acyclovir, valacyclovir, famciclovir or intravenous acyclovir; depending on the disease severity [3].

Varicella zoster virus (VZV) is another human herpes virus and its reactivation typically presents as painful vesicular rash affecting two or less adjacent unilateral dermatomes. The prevalence of herpes zoster has largely declined since the introduction of VZV vaccines. In this case, clinically the lesions were painful; diagnostics revealed absence of VZV on PCR testing of skin swab, which excluded herpes zoster infection [15].

Impetigo is an acute gram-positive bacterial infection of the superficial layers of the epidermis. It presents with pruritus and honey crusted vesicles and erosions around the mouth, nose and other exposed parts of the body, sparing the palms and soles. It is highly contagious and is most prevalent in children between the age of 2–5 years of age, but can occur at any age. Diagnosis of impetigo is usually made clinically. Impetigo was excluded in our case because the vesicles did not have typical honey-crust appearance and were painful rather than pruritic. Clinical diagnosis of impetigo can be confirmed with Gram stain and culture, if in doubt [7, 13].

Cellulitis is an infection causing acute and non-suppurative inflammation of the dermis and subcutaneous fat. On the other hand, abscess is a complication of cellulitis, where neutrophils accumulate in the inflamed tissue to form a collection of pus. On sonography, cellulitis typically presents as diffused thickening of the skin and subcutaneous tissues with a 'cobblestone' appearance of hypoechoic strands of oedematous fluid between connective tissues and the hyperechoic fat. This is different from classical abscess, which presents as an anechoic or hypoechoic focalised fluid collection with irregular or lobulated borders. Gentle pressure can be applied to the queried site using the transducer and resultant movement or "swirling" can verify liquefied abscess [1].

MRSA colonisation in hospitalised dermatology patients have been reported to be as high as 45 %, through both nosocomial and community acquisition. Patients with pemphigus and other bullous diseases are most commonly affected, in a prospective study of a tertiary hospital in Brazil [12]. The Clinical Practice Guidelines by the Infectious Diseases Society of America recommends incision and drainage, as the primary management for cutaneous abscess, and additional antibiotics in immunosuppressed patients while the culture result is pending. Possible empirical therapy includes clindamycin and trimethoprim-sulfamethoxazole. In complicated cases involving deeper soft-tissue infections, wound infections, major abscesses, cellulitis and infected ulcers and burns; intravenous (IV) vancomycin, oral or IV linezolid 600 mg twice daily, daptomycin 4 mg/kg/dose IV once daily, telavancin 10 mg/kg/dose IV once daily, and clindamycin 600 mg IV or PO 3 times a day are recommended empirical therapy for MRSA in addition to broad-spectrum antibiotics and surgical debridement [11].

Skin hygiene, antimicrobial wash, antiseptic dressings on open wounds are some strategies to prevent bacterial impetiginisation. Antimicrobial prophylaxis, such as penicillin V 25 mg twice daily or erythromycin 250 mg twice daily could be used in highly susceptible groups. Antiviral prophylaxis against HSV is also available, along with prophylactic antifungal therapies. When contraindications are not present, patients should be immunised with HZV vaccine and be educated about early signs and symptoms of infections and the need to seek medical advice [10].

Key Points

- Secondary skin infections and systemic infection should be checked in patients with autoimmune blistering conditions.
- HSV infection is associated with PV relapse and in PV patients who become unresponsive to immunosuppressive therapy. Typical presentations include larger lesions, deeper ulceration, delayed wound healing and satellite lesions.
- Classical liquefied abscess presents as an anechoic or hypoechoic focal fluid collection with irregular or lobulated borders on ultrasound. Primary management for cutaneous abscess is incision and drainage and additional antibiotics should be given in immunosuppressed patients while the culture result is pending.

References

1. Adhikari S, Blaivas M. Sonography first for subcutaneous abscess and cellulitis evaluation. J Ultrasound Med. 2012;31(10):1509–12.
2. Amagai M. (2008) Pemphigus. In: H. T, Callen JP, Mancini AJ, et al., (Ed). Dermatology, (2 ed., vol. 1). St. Louis, MO: Elsevier
3. Brady RC, Bernstein DI. Treatment of herpes simplex virus infections. Antiviral Res. 2004;61(2):73–81. doi:http://dx.doi.org/10.1016/j.antiviral.2003.09.006
4. Brandao ML, Fernandes NC, Batista DP, Santos N. Refractory pemphigus vulgaris associated with herpes infection: case report and review. Rev Inst Med Trop Sao Paulo. 2011;53(2):113–7.
5. Caldarola G, Kneisel A, Hertl M, Feliciani C. Herpes simplex virus infection in pemphigus vulgaris: clinical and immunological considerations. Eur J Dermatol. 2008;18(4):440–3. doi:http://dx.doi.org/10.1684/ejd.2008.0439
6. Cheng HF, Lam MS, Tsang KH, Ho WC, Ng WF, Kwan WK. Pemphigus foliaceus complicated by disseminated cutaneous herpes simplex virus infection in an elderly man. Hong Kong J Dermatol Venereol. 2013;21:73–7.

7. Cole C, Gazewood J. Diagnosis and treatment of impetigo. Am Fam Physician. 2007;75(6):859–64.
8. Esmaili N, Mortazavi H, Noormohammadpour P, Boreiri M, Soori T, Vasheghani Farahani I, Mohit M. Pemphigus vulgaris and infections: a retrospective study on 155 patients. Autoimmun Dis. 2013;5. doi:10.1155/2013/834295.
9. Lecluse ALY, Bruijnzeel-Koomen CAFM. Herpes simplex virus infection mimicking bullous disease in an immunocompromised patient. Case Rep Dermatol. 2010;2(2):99–102.
10. Lehman JS, Khunger M, Lohse CM. Infection in autoimmune bullous diseases: a retrospective comparative study. J Dermatol. 2013;40(8):613–9. doi:10.1111/1346-8138.12175.
11. Liu C, Bayer A, Cosgrove SE, Daum RS, Fridkin SK, Gorwitz RJ . . . Chambers HF. Clinical practice guidelines by the infectious diseases society of America for the treatment of methicillin-resistant Staphylococcus aureus infections in adults and children: executive summary. Clin Infect Dis. 2011;52(3):285–92. doi:10.1093/cid/cir034.
12. Pacheco RL, Lobo RD, Oliveira MS, Farina EF, Santos CR, Costa SF . . . Levin AS. Methicillin-resistant Staphylococcus aureus (MRSA) carriage in a dermatology unit. Clinics (Sao Paulo). 2011;66(12):2071–7.
13. Wolff K, Johnson RA, Suurmond D. Bacterial infections involving the skin. In: Wolff K, Johnson RA, Suurmond D, ed. Fitzpatrick's Color Atlas & Synopsis of Clinical Dermatology, ed 6. New York: McGraw-Hill; 2009.
14. Wysocki AB. Evaluating and managing open skin wounds: colonization versus infection. AACN Clin Issues. 2002;13(3):382–97.
15. Zuckerman RA, Limaye AP. Varicella Zoster Virus (VZV) and Herpes Simplex Virus (HSV) in solid organ transplant patients. Am J Transplant. 2013;13:55–66. doi:10.1111/ajt.12003.

Chapter 12
A 57 Year Old Woman with Widespread Scales and Scattered Erosions

Cathy Y. Zhao and Dédée F. Murrell

In November 2010, a 59-year-old female of Indonesian background presented with a 3 year history of a deteriorating and widespread scaly rash. She has no other medical history and had been on no medications. She reported her rash had been diagnosed as "eczema" and could not recall how her rash initially developed. On examination, she had an exfoliative erythroderma with thick scales over her face, trunk, hands and feet (Figs. 12.1, 12.2, and 12.3). Amongst the scales there were several shallow erosions. Her palms and feet were hyperkeratotic. However her mucosal membranes were spared. On further questioning, it was found that she had had skin biopsies taken from her arms and cheek for the same

C.Y. Zhao, M.B.B.S., MMed
Department of Dermatology, St George Hospital,
Level 0, James Laws House, Gray Street, Kogarah,
Sydney, NSW 2217, Australia

D.F. Murrell, M.A., BMBCh, FAAD, M.D., FACD (✉)
Department of Dermatology, St George Hospital,
Level 0, James Laws House, Gray Street, Kogarah,
Sydney, NSW 2217, Australia

University of New South Wales, Sydney, NSW Australia
e-mail: d.murrell@unsw.edu.au

D.F. Murrell (ed.), *Clinical Cases in Autoimmune
Blistering Diseases*, Clinical Cases in Dermatology 5,
DOI 10.1007/978-3-319-10148-4_12,
© Springer International Publishing Switzerland 2015

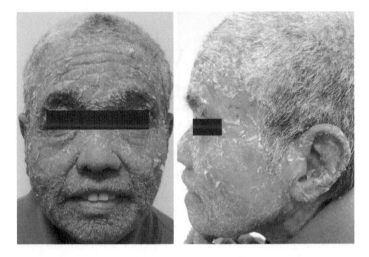

FIGURE 12.1 Scales over the patient's face, ears and scalp with perioral and periorbital crusts

problem at another dermatology institution in 2008. Retrieval of the biopsy report revealed focal superficial acantholysis in the subcorneal zone with parakeratosis and hyperkeratosis. Direct immunofluorescence was negative but indirect immunofluorescence showed intercellular IgG in the epidermis, including at the surface. A diagnosis was made with the combination of clinical presentation, histopathology and immunofluorescence in 2008. However as the patient had been lost to follow-up, she was not informed of her diagnosis nor had been on any treatments for it. A repeat biopsy for direct immunofluorescence was positive between the keratinocytes for IgG.

Based on the case description and the photograph, what is your diagnosis?

1. Pityriasis rubra pilaris
2. Pemphigus foliaceus
3. Ichthyosis
4. IgA pemphigus

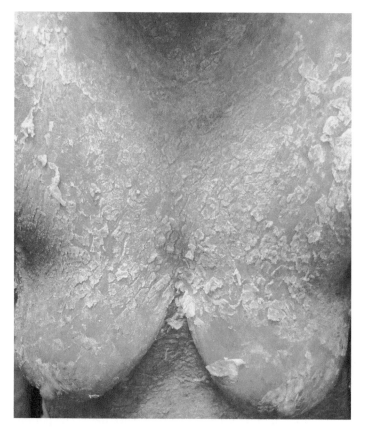

FIGURE 12.2 Exfoliative scales covering the patient's chest

Diagnosis

Pemphigus Foliaceus

The patient was diagnosed with pemphigus foliaceus (PF) and immediately hospitalised. Due to her age and concern for an initial possible infection, systemic treatment began with a course of prednisone starting at 25 mg daily for 1 month and,

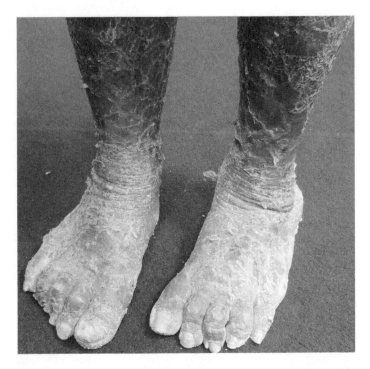

FIGURE 12.3 Scales over the patient's legs and feet with dystrophic toe nails

after a normal G6PD, dapsone 50 mg twice daily. The patient responded well with her blisters resolving. However, in February 2011, her haemoglobin dropped to 104 with reticulocyte of 235, consistent with dapsone-induced haemolysis. Hence her dapsone was ceased.

The patient remained stable for 3 months until May 2011, when her PF relapsed and became resistant to treatment. New blisters and erosions developed over her scalp, arms and upper trunk (Fig. 12.2). Her anti-Dsg 1 level was 250 U/ml (normal <20). This relapse coincided with her being started on perindopril by her family doctor, a well-known cause of PF, which was then ceased and changed to metoprolol. Without the dapsone, her PF was a challenge as it did not respond to multiple other treatment modalities over the next 18 months. These treatments included azathioprine 100 mg twice daily, fixed-dose prednisone of up to 70 mg daily (1 mg/kg/day), IVIG infusions monthly and four weekly doses of 375 mg/m^2 rituximab.

In January 2012, as her PF remained active, further treatment modalities were trialed with minimal response. She was commenced on mycophenolate 750 mg twice daily as an alternative to azathioprine, and methotrexate gradually increased to 17.5 mg daily while her prednisone was tapered. However, her PF remained active despite the above with PDAI (Pemphigus Disease Area Index) activity score of up to 65.

In April 2013, the patient was recommenced on low dose dapsone and her PF improved. Although she previously had haemolysis with dapsone, it was the only medication her PF had responded to. Her dapsone was recommenced at a small dose of 25 mg weekly, gradually increased to five times weekly over the next 6 months. Her haemoglobin and reticulocyte count were monitored fortnightly, which remained stable. With a combination of dapsone, IVIG infusions, tapered prednisone, mycophenalate and methotrexate, her lesions finally reduced in severity and quantity by end of 2013. Eventually her PF was in remission, and was maintained on dapsone 25 mg five times weekly, tapered prednisone decreased to 6 mg daily and IVIG infusions monthly. Her anti dsg1 ELISA is now 150 U/ml with PDAI of 16.

Discussion

Pemphigus foliaceus (PF) is an acquired autoimmune blistering disease, and accounts for approximately 10 % of all cases of the pemphigus group but may vary in some countries which have an endemic form of PF [8]. It is characterised by the immune system producing auto-antibodies of mainly IgG4 subclass that target the intercellular adhesion glycoprotein desmoglein 1 (Dsg 1). The main two subtypes of PF are idiopathic PF, which is found universally and occurs sporadically, and endemic PF known as *fogo selvagem*, which occurs in certain geographical areas.

The diagnosis of PF requires three criteria: clinical presentation, histopathology and the presence of auto-antibodies as detected by either direct immunofluorescence (DIF) or indirect immunofluorescence (IIF). Regarding its clinical presentation, PF commonly begin on the trunk, before spreading. Its primary lesions are flaccid, superficial blisters which easily rupture and hence are often missed by clinicians. Commonly, only secondary lesions such as erosions and crusts are observed. The severest form of PF can produce an exfoliative erythroderma. It typically does not affect mucosal surfaces including the oral cavity. It is important to be aware that early PF may mimic various other scaly conditions, causing delays of up to years in making the correct diagnosis. Clinicians should always enquire about the primary lesions in scaly and erosive diseases to try illicit the history of blistering which is not always possible. As our patient did not recall a history of blisters, she was initially misdiagnosed as eczema. Other differential diagnoses of PF include drug eruptions, IgA pemphigus, lupus erythematosus, ichthyosis, psoriasis, pityriasis rubra pilaris and Darier's disease.

Histopathology of PF lesions manifests differently according to stages of disease progression. Early PF lesions show vacuoles in the intercellular spaces of the upper epidermis and established PF lesions show blisters in the subcorneal zone or high in the granular layer [6]. Meanwhile, older PF lesions show evidence of chronic inflammation including papillomatosis, acantholysis, parakeratosis, hyperkeratosis and follicular plugging, consistent with our patient [3]. The DIF and IIF of PF have sensitivities of 80–95 % and 79–90 %, respectively, and are characterised by an intercellular space staining pattern, likely more intense in the upper epidermis [1, 4].

Our case also highlights the importance of performing a thorough medication review in PF, as multiple drugs have been found to be associated with the development of it. These include disease modifying anti-rheumatic drugs such as penicillamine and bucillamine, ACE (angiotensin-converting enzyme) inhibitors, angiotensin-II receptor blockers, rifampicin and tiopronin. Other than oral medications, ultraviolet light and ionising radiation may also induce or exacerbate PF [5]. Our patient's PF relapse of in May 2011 is likely induced by her commencement of perindopril, an ACE inhibitor.

The treatment modalities for PF are many including systemic glucocorticoids, immunosuppressive therapies and anti-inflammatory therapies. Treatment choice can be complex as patient co-morbidities, compliance, risk profile and cost must be considered. There is evidence for systemic glucocorticoids being central to the effective management of PF, although there is no evidence suggesting a specific dose or regime. Many experts suggest 1 mg/kg/day but this would need to be weighed against the risk profile and efficacy of the glucocorticoid in the specific patient [7]. In our patient, higher dose prednisone of 70 mg (1 mg/kg/day) was not as effective as low-dose prednisone at 20 mg daily combined with dapsone.

Various immunosuppressive and anti-inflammatory therapies all have evidence supporting a steroid-supporting role, however, limited evidence for PF remission or maintenance [2]. Immunosuppressive therapies used include azathioprine, mycophenolate mofetil, methotrexate, cyclophosphamide and cyclosporine. Anti-inflammatory therapies used include dapsone, IVIG and plasmapheresis. These therapies need to be carefully monitored when prescribed as each may be associated with serious side effects (Table 12.1).

Our case illustrates the complexity of choosing the most suitable therapy regimen. Like our patient, PF at times can be very drug-resistant and multiple immunosuppressive and anti-inflammatory therapies in adjunct to systemic glucocorticoids may need to be trialed before finding the most effective regimen. Also, like the dapsone in our case, a flexible approach may need to be taken when patients experience side effects to the effective therapy, such as recommencing the medication at a lower dose. The patient's haemolysis while on dapsone 50 mg daily resolved when her dapsone dose was reduced to 25 mg 5 days weekly.

TABLE 12.1 Immunosuppressive and anti-inflammatory therapies for PF, administration and side effects (Frew et al [2])

Therapy	Administration	Side effects
Azathioprine	Oral: usually 100–200 mg per day	Myelosuppression, nausea, hepatotoxicity
Mycophenolate mofetil	Oral: up to 2–3 g per day	Neutropenia, lymphopenia, anaemia, thrombocytopenia, nausea
Cyclophosphamide	Intravenous or oral	Neutropenia, nausea, hepatotoxicity
Cyclosporine	Oral	Hypertension, renal impairment, nausea
Methotrexate	Oral	Myelosuppresion, hepatotoxicity, pulmonary fibrosis
Dapsone	Oral	Haemolysis, methaemoglobinaemia
Intravenous immunoglobulin	IV	Infusion reaction, anaphylaxis
Plasmapheresis	IV	Septicaemia, electrolyte disturbances

Key Points

Pemphigus foliaceus can mimic various other scaly or crusty conditions, causing delays in diagnosis.

Histopathology of PF lesions manifests differently according to stages of disease progression.

Multiple drugs are found to be associated with the development of pemphigus foliaceus.

The treatment modalities for PF are many and treatment choice can be complex.

References

1. Bystryn JC, Abel FL, DeFeo D. Pemphigus foliaceus: subcorneal intercellular antibodies of unique specificity. Arch Dermatol. 1974;110:857–61.
2. Frew JW, Martin LK, Murrell DF. Evidence-based treatments in pemphigus vulgaris and pemphigus foliaceus. Dermatol Clin. 2011;29(4):599–606.
3. Furtado TA. Histopathology of pemphigus foliaceus. AMA Arch Dermatol. 1959;80(1):66–71.
4. Harrist TJ, Mihm Jr MC. Cutaneous immunopathology. The diagnostic use of direct and indirect immunofluorescence techniques in diagnostic dermatopathology. Hum Pathol. 1979;10:625.
5. James KA, Culton DA, Diaz LA. Diagnosis and clinical features of pemphigus foliaceus. Dermatol Clin. 2011;29(3):405–12.
6. Kouskoukis CE, Ackerman AB. What histologic finding distinguishes superficial pemphigus and bullous impetigo? Am J Dermatopathol. 1984;6:179–81.
7. Murrell DF, Dick S, Ahmed AR, et al. Consensus statement on definitions of disease, end points and therapeutic response for pemphigus. J Am Acad Dermatol. 2008;58:1043–6.
8. Ryan JG. Pemphigus. A 20-year survey of experience with 70 cases. Arch Dermatol. 1971;104:14–20.

Chapter 13
Pemphigus Foliaceus, var. Herpetiformis and Sulphonamide

Valeria Aoki and Denise Miyamoto

A 43-year-old woman presented a 2-year history of tender blisters and erythematous and crusted excoriations on the face, trunk and proximal extremities. During her first examination in 1995, erosions and yellow crusts on her face, thorax, upper torso and proximal limbs were present, without mucosal involvement. Laboratory profile confirmed the diagnosis of pemphigus foliaceus, as follows: histopathological analysis exhibited subcorneal abscess with mild spongiosis and scanty acantholytic cells; neutrophilic and linfohystiocitic perivascular infiltrate was present in the superficial dermis; direct immunofluorescence showed intercellular IgG deposits within the entire epidermis; indirect immunofluorescence revealed circulating IgG antibodies (titer=1:1,280) and positive ELISA index (99, recombinant desmoglein 1). Treatment with systemic corticosteroid (prednisone 1 mg/kg/day) was initiated. Clinical remission was achieved after 2 months, followed by gradual corticosteroid tapering. The patient presented reactivation when receiving prednisone 10 mg/day, with vesicles with a herpetiform arrangement on erythematous plaques on her legs, with intense pruritus (Fig. 13.1).

V. Aoki, M.D., Ph.D. (✉) • D. Miyamoto, M.D.
Immunodermatology Laboratory, Department of Dermatology, University of Sao Paulo Medical School, São Paulo, Brazil
e-mail: valeria.aoki@gmail.com

D.F. Murrell (ed.), *Clinical Cases in Autoimmune Blistering Diseases*, Clinical Cases in Dermatology 5, DOI 10.1007/978-3-319-10148-4_13, © Springer International Publishing Switzerland 2015

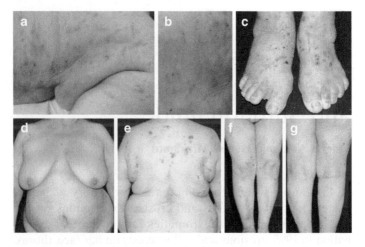

FIGURE 13.1 Pemphigus foliaceus (var.) herpetiformis: (**a, b**) grouped vesicles, bullae and crusts over erythematous and edematous plaques on torso and (**c**) dorsal aspect of the feet, (**d**) and (**e**) pruritic vesicles on the trunk and sparse lesions on the inferior limbs (**f**) and (**g**)

Based on the case description and the photograph, what is your diagnosis?

1. Pemphigus foliaceus
2. Pemphigus herpetiformis
3. Dermatitis herpetiformis
4. Bullous pemphigoid
5. Linear IgA bullous dermatosis

After a negative Tzanck smear, a new biopsy was performed, and histopathology analysis showed eosinophilic spongiosis (Fig. 13.2). Immunological studies (Fig. 13.3) revealed intercellular, intraepidermal deposits of IgG and C3, circulating IgG antibodies (titer 1:320) and maintenance of positive ELISA index for desmoglein 1 (45), consistent with the diagnosis of pemphigus herpetiformis. Prednisone was increased to 30 mg/day, associated to sulfamethoxypyridazine (1 g/day). Lesions rapidly improved after 5 weeks, allowing corticosteroid and sulphonamide discontinuation after 3 months. She presented new lesions 1 month after therapy

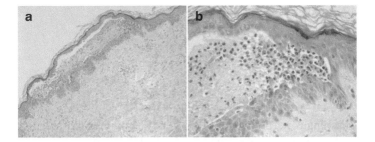

FIGURE 13.2 Pemphigus foliaceus (var.) herpetiformis: (a) intraepidermal cleavage with acantholytic cells in the upper layers; (b) scanty acantholysis with adjacent eosinophilic spongiosis

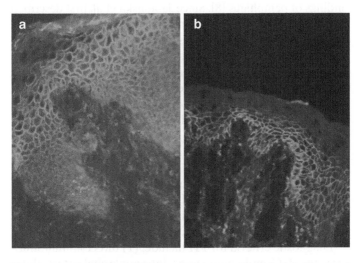

FIGURE 13.3 Pemphigus foliaceus (var.) herpetiformis: (a) direct and (b) indirect immunofluorescence showing intense intercellular IgG deposits within the epidermis

was withdrawn, and prednisone 40 mg/day and sulfamethoxypyridazine 1 g/day were reintroduced. Partial remission occurred after 4 months, and due to sporadic erythematous, pruritic papules and plaques on the trunk, sulphonamide was administered to the patient for 10 years.

Diagnosis

Pemphigus foliaceus (var. herpetiformis)

Discussion

Pemphigus herpetiformis (PH) is an uncommon intraepidermal autoimmune blistering disease with incidence rates up to 7.3 % among pemphigus patients [15]. This rare variant of pemphigus shows no gender predilection [15, 17, 24], and is predominantly observed in adults [22]. PH exhibits clinical features similar to dermatitis herpetiformis and immunological findings of pemphigus [8]. Since Jablonska et al. first described PH in 1975, nearly 100 cases have been reported [10].

Clinical presentation consists of pruritic vesicles, papules and bullae over erythematous background, arranged in a herpetiform distribution. Some lesions may centrifugally spread, originating annular and polycyclic plaques [22]. Usual sites of involvement are the thorax, torso, and proximal limbs; mucous membranes are usually spared [19, 22]. Differential diagnosis include pemphigus foliaceus, pemphigus vulgaris, bullous pemphigoid, linear IgA bullous dermatosis and dermatitis herpetiformis [6].

Similar to its polymorphous clinical features, histopathologic findings are variable [22], showing spongiosis with eosinophils and/or neutrophils, microabscesses and blister formation, with mild or no evident acantholysis [8, 10, 22].

Diagnostic criteria for PH include: (1) direct immunofluorescence: IgG and complement intraepidermal intercellular deposits [10, 22, 24]; (2) indirect immunofluorescence: circulating IgG antibodies against desmosome components [10, 22, 24]; (3) enzyme-linked immunosorbent assay: anti-desmoglein 1 circulating antibodies (also consider anti-desmoglein 3 and anti-desmocollin 3) [10, 11, 22].

PH pathogenesis remains unclear. Santi et al. reported seven cases of PH in which two patients developed lesions before pemphigus foliaceus (n=1) and pemphigus vulgaris (n=1) diagnosis, and five patients who presented lesions consistent with PH during PF (n=4) and PV treatment (n=1). Therefore, PH could be a transient, clinical presentation of classical pemphigus [24].

Current evidence suggests the occurrence of an epitope-spreading phenomenon: autoantibodies anti-desmoglein 1 and 3 bind to different antigen sites. Kubo et al. proposed that in pemphigus foliaceus and pemphigus vulgaris, pathogenic IgG autoantibodies disrupt adhesive properties of desmogleins and activate proteinases signaling and release, causing acantholysis. Meanwhile, acantholysis is rarely observed in PH because keratinocyte adhesion mediated by desmogleins is preserved [12]. O'Toole et al. demonstrated that in PH patients, IgG autoantibodies upregulate IL-8 production by keratinocytes, which attracts neutrophils [20]. After recruitment and activation mediated by the Fc portion of IgG, neutrophils secrete proteases leading to spongiosis [10].

IgG subclasses might be another determinant of disease profile. IgG1 and IgG3 are predominant during remission or preclinical asympthomatic pemphigus vulgaris, while IgG4 is a marker of disease activity [2, 25]. Nevertheless, in PH, IgG1 and IgG3, but not IgG4 are able to induce eosinophilic activation and degranulation with release of mediators that promote spongiosis and possibly mild acantholysis [9].

Since neutrophils and eosinophils play an important role in the pathogenesis of PH, dapsone is the first line treatment. Sulphonamide reduces polymorphonuclear chemotaxis, and inhibits tissue damage mediated by lysosomal enzymes and toxic oxygen species [3, 7]. Dosages vary from 100 to 300 mg/day in monotherapy or combined with low dose systemic corticosteroid [1].

PH has a good prognosis with rapid response to therapy in about two thirds of the patients [14], especially when antibody serum titers are low or absent, and eosinophilic spongiosis is observed [1, 5]. As patients with PH may progress to PF or PV, systemic corticosteroid and immunosuppressants should be considered in their treatment [24]. Some cases of PH associated with psoriasis [18, 23], infections [4], neoplasms

[13, 16, 19, 21] and drugs [26, 27] were reported, but due to the rarity of this pemphigus variant, a true correlation remains uncertain.

Key Points

- Pemphigus herpetiformis is a rare pemphigus variant, with clinical features resembling dermatitis herpetiformis and immunological profile consistent with pemphigus
- Prognosis is good, with great response to dapsone therapy
- Pemphigus herpetiformis may be the first clinical presentation and then progress to pemphigus vulgaris or foliaceus, or may arise during treatment of classic forms of pemphigus

References

1. Basset N, Guillot B, Michel B, Meynadier J, Guilhou JJ. Dapsone as initial treatment in superficial pemphigus. Report of nine cases. Arch Dermatol. 1987;123(6):783–5.
2. Bhol K, Natarajan K, Nagarwalla N, Mohimen A, Aoki V, Ahmed AR. Correlation of peptide specificity and IgG subclass with pathogenic and nonpathogenic autoantibodies in pemphigus vulgaris: a model for autoimmunity. Proc Natl Acad Sci U S A. 1995;92(11):5239–43.
3. Booth SA, Moody CE, Dahl MV, Herron MJ, Nelson RD. Dapsone suppresses integrin-mediated neutrophil adherence function. J Invest Dermatol. 1992;98(2):135–40.
4. Bull RH, Fallowfield ME, Marsden RA. Autoimmune blistering diseases associated with HIV infection. Clin Exp Dermatol. 1994;19(1):47–50.
5. Dias M, dos Santos AP, Sousa J, Maya M. Herpetiform pemphigus. J Eur Acad Dermatol Venereol. 1999;12(1):82–5.
6. Duarte IB, Bastazini Jr I, Barreto JA, Carvalho CV, Nunes AJ. Pemphigus herpetiformis in childhood. Pediatr Dermatol. 2010;27(5):488–91. doi:10.1111/j.1525-1470.2010.01256.x.
7. Gurcan HM, Ahmed AR. Efficacy of dapsone in the treatment of pemphigus and pemphigoid: analysis of current data. Am J

Clin Dermatol. 2009;10(6):383–96. doi:10.2165/11310740-000000000-00000.

8. Jablonska S, Chorzelski TP, Beutner EH, Chorzelska J. Herpetiform pemphigus, a variable pattern of pemphigus. Int J Dermatol. 1975;14(5):353–9.

9. Kaneko M, Swanson MC, Gleich GJ, Kita H. Allergen-specific IgG1 and IgG3 through Fc gamma RII induce eosinophil degranulation. J Clin Invest. 1995;95(6):2813–21. doi:10.1172/JCI117986.

10. Kasperkiewicz M, Kowalewski C, Jablonska S. Pemphigus herpetiformis: from first description until now. J Am Acad Dermatol. 2014. doi:10.1016/j.jaad.2013.11.043.

11. Kozlowska A, Hashimoto T, Jarzabek-Chorzelska M, Amagai A, Nagata Y, Strasz Z, Jablonska S. Pemphigus herpetiformis with IgA and IgG antibodies to desmoglein 1 and IgG antibodies to desmocollin 3. J Am Acad Dermatol. 2003;48(1):117–22. doi:10.1067/mjd.2003.23.

12. Kubo A, Amagai M, Hashimoto T, Doi T, Higashiyama M, Hashimoto K, Yoshikawa K. Herpetiform pemphigus showing reactivity with pemphigus vulgaris antigen (desmoglein 3). Br J Dermatol. 1997;137(1):109–13.

13. Kubota Y, Yoshino Y, Mizoguchi M. A case of herpetiform pemphigus associated with lung cancer. J Dermatol. 1994;21(8):609–11.

14. Lebeau S, Muller R, Masouye I, Hertl M, Borradori L. Pemphigus herpetiformis: analysis of the autoantibody profile during the disease course with changes in the clinical phenotype. Clin Exp Dermatol. 2010;35(4):366–72. doi:10.1111/j.1365-2230.2009.03525.x.

15. Maciejowska E, Jablonska S, Chorzelski T. Is pemphigus herpetiformis an entity? Int J Dermatol. 1987;26(9):571–7.

16. Marzano AV, Tourlaki A, Cozzani E, Gianotti R, Caputo R. Pemphigus herpetiformis associated with prostate cancer. J Eur Acad Dermatol Venereol. 2007;21(5):696–8. doi:10.1111/j.1468-3083.2006.01992.x.

17. Micali G, Musumeci ML, Nasca MR. Epidemiologic analysis and clinical course of 84 consecutive cases of pemphigus in eastern Sicily. Int J Dermatol. 1998;37(3):197–200.

18. Morita E, Amagai M, Tanaka T, Horiuchi K, Yamamoto S. A case of herpetiform pemphigus coexisting with psoriasis vulgaris. Br J Dermatol. 1999;141(4):754–5.

19. Nakashima H, Fujimoto M, Watanabe R, Ishiura N, Yamamoto AI, Hashimoto T, Tamaki K. Herpetiform pemphigus without

anti-desmoglein 1/3 autoantibodies. J Dermatol. 2010;37(3): 264–8. doi:10.1111/j.1346-8138.2009.00786.x.

20. O'Toole EA, Mak LL, Guitart J, Woodley DT, Hashimoto T, Amagai M, Chan LS. Induction of keratinocyte IL-8 expression and secretion by IgG autoantibodies as a novel mechanism of epidermal neutrophil recruitment in a pemphigus variant. Clin Exp Immunol. 2000;119(1):217–24.

21. Palleschi GM, Giomi B. Herpetiformis pemphigus and lung carcinoma: a case of paraneoplastic pemphigus. Acta Derm Venereol. 2002;82(4):304–5.

22. Robinson ND, Hashimoto T, Amagai M, Chan LS. The new pemphigus variants. J Am Acad Dermatol. 1999;40(5 Pt 1):649–71; quiz 672-643.

23. Sanchez-Palacios C, Chan LS. Development of pemphigus herpetiformis in a patient with psoriasis receiving UV-light treatment. J Cutan Pathol. 2004;31(4):346–9.

24. Santi CG, Maruta CW, Aoki V, Sotto MN, Rivitti EA, Diaz LA. Pemphigus herpetiformis is a rare clinical expression of nonendemic pemphigus foliaceus, fogo selvagem, and pemphigus vulgaris. Cooperative Group on Fogo Selvagem Research. J Am Acad Dermatol. 1996;34(1):40–6.

25. Spaeth S, Riechers R, Borradori L, Zillikens D, Budinger L, Hertl M. IgG, IgA and IgE autoantibodies against the ectodomain of desmoglein 3 in active pemphigus vulgaris. Br J Dermatol. 2001;144(6):1183–8.

26. Verdier-Sevrain S, Joly P, Thomine E, Belanyi P, Gilbert D, Tron F, Lauret P. Thiopronine-induced herpetiform pemphigus: report of a case studied by immunoelectron microscopy and immunoblot analysis. Br J Dermatol. 1994;130(2):238–40.

27. Weltfriend S, Ingber A, David M, Sandbank M. Pemphigus herpetiformis following D-penicillamine in a patient with HLA B8. Der Hautarzt; Zeitschrift fur Dermatologie, Venerologie, und verwandte Gebiete. 1988;39(9):587–8.

Chapter 14
A 43 Year Old with Vegetative Plaques and Erosions on the Trunk

Donna A. Culton and Luis A. Diaz

A 43 year old African American female presented with a 1 year history of pruritic scaly plaques on her scalp. In the 2 months prior to presentation she had begun to develop thick painful vegetative plaques on her scalp as well as her trunk. She denied any history of mucosal lesions concurrently or prior to the cutaneous eruption.

On examination, she was noted to have multiple large vegetative plaques on her scalp, presacral region, abdomen and inframammary folds along with deep erosions within the vegetative plaques (Fig. 14.1a).

Based on the case description and the clinical image, what is your diagnosis?

1. Pemphigus foliaceus
2. Mucosal predominant pemphigus vulgaris

D.A. Culton, M.D., Ph.D. (✉) • L.A. Diaz
Department of Dermatology, University of North Carolina at Chapel Hill, 401 Mary Ellen Jones Bldg, CB#7287,
Chapel Hill, NC 27599, USA
e-mail: culton@med.unc.edu

D.F. Murrell (ed.), *Clinical Cases in Autoimmune Blistering Diseases*, Clinical Cases in Dermatology 5, DOI 10.1007/978-3-319-10148-4_14,
© Springer International Publishing Switzerland 2015

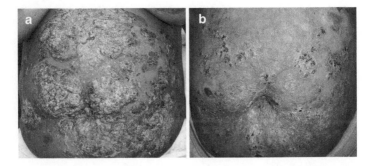

FIGURE 14.1 Clinical findings at the time of presentation with large vegetative plaques with deep erosions over the abdomen (**a**) that were significantly improved 2 weeks after treatment with a single cycle of IVIg (**b**)

3. Mucocutaneous pemphigus vulgaris
4. Cutaneous pemphigus vulgaris
5. Bullous pemphigoid

Biopsy for routine histology revealed suprabasilar clefting with numerous acantholytic keratinocytes with prominent extension down follicular epithelium. Biopsy for direct immunofluorescence showed deposition of IgG in the intracellular spaces (ICS) of the epidermis. Indirect immunofluorescence was positive with IgG reactivity in the ICS spaces of monkey esophagus at a final titer of 1:640. Anti-desmoglein (Dsg) 1 and Dsg3 ELISA studies revealed index values of 163.4 and 119.4, respectively (normal range <20U).

At the time of presentation, she was failing prednisone 80 mg daily. She was treated with 1 cycle of intravenous immunoglobulin (IVIg) and azathioprine was added as a steroid sparing agent. Two weeks following IVIg she showed significant clinical improvement (Fig 14.1b). Her prednisone was successfully tapered and she was controlled on azathioprine as monotherapy.

Diagnosis

Cutaneous pemphigus vulgaris

Discussion

Pemphigus vulgaris (PV) is a group of autoimmune blistering disorders mediated by autoantibodies against the desomosomal adhesion proteins Dsg1 and Dsg3. Three distinct clinical forms of PV have been described (Table 14.1):

Mucosal predominant PV (mPV) is characterized clinically by mucosal erosions that most commonly affect the oral mucosa, but can also involve the nasal and genital mucosa as well. Routine histology shows suprabasilar clefting and acantholysis. Direct immunofluorescence (DIF) shows deposition of IgG at the ICS spaces throughout the epidermis. Indirect immunofluorescence (IIF) confirms circulating IgG with reactivity to the ICS spaces with monkey esophagus as the preferred substrate. The autoantibodies in mPV are limited to Dsg3 specificity alone. Interestingly, many pemphigus

TABLE 14.1 Histological and immunological findings in pemphigus variants

	Mucosal PV	**Mucocuta-neous PV**	**Cutaneous PV**	**Pemphigus foliaceus (PF)**
H&E	Suprabasilar cleft	Suprabasilar cleft	Suprabasilar cleft	Subcorneal cleft
Site(s) involved	Mucosa	Mucosa	------	------
	------	Skin	Skin	Skin
Antigenic target(s)	Dsg3	Dsg3	Dsg3	------
	------	Dsg1	Dsg1	Dsg1

patients recall lesions limited to the mucosal surfaces at the onset of their disease. While some patients remain with lesions limited to the mucosa for the duration of their disease and are eventually categorized as mPV, most patients progress to mucocutaneous PV [1, 3].

Mucocutaneous PV (mcPV) is the most common form of PV. Clinically, patients show flaccid bullae and erosions involving the mucosa as well as the skin. Vegetative plaques may be present and in these cases, the term pemphigus vegetans may be used. Routine histology and immunofluorescence features are similar to those described in mPV above, however extension of suprabasilar clefting and acantholysis often extends down the follicular epithelium when hair bearing skin is involved. The autoantibodies in mcPV recognize not only Dsg3 (as in mPV), but Dsg1 as well [1, 3].

Cutaneous PV (cPV) is a relatively newly described and rare form of PV. Clinically, cPV patients have lesions limited to the skin. The lack of mucosal involvement distinguishes cPV from mcPV described above. The clinical features can be quite variable with reports of pemphigus foliaceus (see below), vesicular pemphigoid (see below), and classic PV type lesions on the skin [5–8]. The diagnosis is confirmed by histology showing suprabasilar clefting and acantholysis. DIF and IIF findings are identical to those seen in mcPV. The autoantibodies in cPV recognize both Dsg1 and Dsg3 as in mcPV, with higher index values for anti-Dsg1 antibodies. Some authors reserve the designation of cPV for patients with lack of mucosal lesions throughout the duration of their disease. However, transition from mcPV to cPV has also been described [4, 8]. In these cases, transition to cPV is marked by a relative decrease in the anti-Dsg3 index values.

Pemphigus foliaceus (PF) is another autoimmune blistering disorder in the pemphigus family. In contrast to mPV and mcPV, but similar to cPV, PF patients have lesions restricted to the skin. However, histology of PF shows subcorneal clefting and acantholysis (as opposed to suprabasilar involvement seen in PV). Given the superficial nature of the clefting, clinical findings often include superficial erosions and scaling as opposed to intact blisters. DIF findings are similar to those described for PV with IgG deposition in ICS spaces. IIF shows IgG reactivity to the ICS spaces with normal human skin being the preferred substrate. The autoantibodies in PF are limited to Dsg1 specificity [3].

Bullous pemphigoid is also an autoimmune blistering disorder that involves the skin. It most often occurs in the elderly population and is associated with significant pruritus. While there are some variants that can affect the mucosa, the classic form of bullous pemphigoid presents with tense bullae overlying urticarial plaques limited to the skin. Histology reveals subepidermal clefting with a dermal infiltrate of eosinophils along with neutrophils and lymphocytes. DIF shows C3 and IgG in a linear staining pattern along the basement membrane. IIF shows IgG localizing to the epidermal side of the salt split skin substrate. These findings are the result of autoantibodies against the NC16A domain of the hemidesmosomal protein BP180 [2].

Though the patient described in this case only had cutaneous lesions as is frequently seen in PF, the suprabasilar clefting on histology and the presence of both anti-Dsg1 and Dsg3 autoantibodies by ELISA confirmed a diagnosis of cPV. The vegetative nature of the plaques were consistent with a pemphigus vegetans morphology. Though not a previously described clinical presentation of cPV, the pemphigus vegetans morphology is more commonly a feature of pemphigus vulgaris and this finding was also supportive of the diagnosis of cPV.

Key Points

- Cutaneous pemphigus vulgaris shows classic findings of pemphigus, but lacks mucosal lesions on exam or by history.
- Diagnosis relies on histologic findings of suprabasilar clefting and acantholysis and confirmatory immunofluorescence findings of IgG deposition in ICS staining pattern.
- ELISA shows antibodies to both Dsg1 and Dsg3.

References

1. Ding X, Aoki V, Mascaro Jr JM, Lopez-Swiderski A, Diaz LA, Fairley JA. Mucosal and mucocutaneous (generalized) pemphigus vulgaris show distinct autoantibody profiles. J Invest Dermatol. 1997;109:592–6.
2. Di Zenzo G, della Torre R, Zambruno G, Borradori L. Bullous pemphigoid: from the clinic to the bench. Clin Dermatol. 2012;30: 3–16.
3. Joly P, Litrowski N. Pemphigus group (vulgaris, vegetans, foliaceus, herpetiformis, brasiliensis). Clin Dermatol. 2011;29:423–36.
4. Matsuda-Hirose H, Ishikawa K, Goto M, Hatano Y, Fujiwara S. Selective elevation of antibodies to desmoglein 1 during the transition from mucocutaneous to cutaneous type pemphigus vulgaris. Ann Dermatol. 2013;25(2):263–5.
5. Muller E, Kernland K, Caldelari R, Wyder M, Balmer V, Hunziker T. Unusual pemphigus phenotype in the presence of a Dsg1 and Dsg3 autoantibody profile. J Invest Dermatol. 2002;118:551–5.
6. Nagasaka A, Matsue H, Miyahara A, Shimada S. Pemphigus vulgaris with no mucosal lesions showing pemphigus-foliaceus-like skin manifestations. Is there a 'cutaneous type' of pemphigus vulgaris? Dermatology. 2005;211:372–4.
7. Shinkuma S, Nishie W, Shibaki A, Sawamura D, Ito K, Tsuji-Abe Y, Natsuga K, Chan PT, Amagai M, Shimizu H. Cutaneous pemphigus vulgaris with skin features similar to the classic mucocutaneous type: a case report and review of the literature. Clin Exp Dermatol. 2008;33:724–8.
8. Yoshida K, Takae Y, Saito H, Oka H, Tanikawa A, Amagai M, Nishikawa T. Cutaneous type pemphigus vulgaris: a rare clinical phenotype of pemphigus. J Am Acad Dermatol. 2005;52:839–45.

Chapter 15
Dermatitis Herpetiformis

Sarolta Kárpáti

A 2.5 Year Old Small Boy with Itchy Skin Symptoms Treated for Atopic Dermatitis

The 2.5 year old boy presented with an itchy skin rash above the elbows, knees and buttocks. He had been treated for atopic dermatitis, but did not improve. Since the distribution of the symptoms suggested dermatitis herpetiformis (DH), we performed immunofluorescence from the perilesional skin and could confirm the diagnosis by the characteristic IgA staining in the dermal papilla (Fig. 15.1) and by the endomysium antibody (EMA) positivity, diagnostic for celiac disease (CD) (that time no transglutaminase (TG) 2 or 3 ELISAs were available) [1]. He also underwent a small bowel biopsy by Crosby capsule and showed mild partial villous atrophy and a pathologic IgA staining in the jejunum [2]-today recognized as TG2 bound IgA staining- and was treated by gluten free diet (GFD) and by low dose dapsone. While there were no laboratory side effects from the drug detected, his steps became uncertain, and could not run as

S. Kárpáti
Department of Dermatology, Venereology and Dermatooncology,
Semmelweis University, Budapest, Hungary
e-mail: skarpati@t-online.hu

D.F. Murrell (ed.), *Clinical Cases in Autoimmune Blistering Diseases*, Clinical Cases in Dermatology 5, DOI 10.1007/978-3-319-10148-4_15, © Springer International Publishing Switzerland 2015

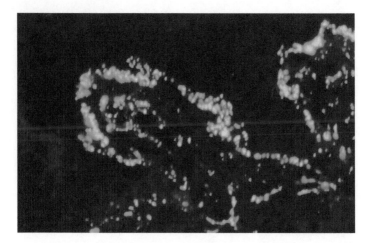

FIGURE 15.1 IgA granules within the papillary dermis

before. When we stopped the medication his movement recovered. He went on solely with the GFD and his skin became symptom-free. Several years later the patient's father developed severe weight loss and was treated for anorexia nervosa. He asked us whether we could check him for CD, since he did not feel the psychological urge to hunger, but suffered from recurrent diarrhea. He was diagnosed with an acute CD. That time, his other son was also investigated for gluten sensitivity and he was also EMA positive, and had mild partial villous atrophy on jejunal biopsy. The mother was not affected by the disease, and none of the family members had associated diseases at that time.

Key Points to Case 1

1. DH can develop at any age, rarely in the very young, or in very elderly too
2. Dapsone can induce temporary neuropathies, mostly in the older age group, and, as in this case, in the very young, too
3. Screening of immediate family members of DH patients for CD is necessary

A Young Male with "Well Treated", Symptom-Free Celiac Disease Developed an Itchy, Crusted Skin Rash

This patient had a long history of coeliac disease (CD). The boy was diagnosed with acute CD within his first year of life and was treated by gluten-free diet (GFD) by the pediatric gastroenterology department. He had no further major medical problems before puberty when he felt unwell and different, and started to eat some gluten containing food when he was with friends or joined to companies. Although he was controlled for the CD, and he did not have clinical symptoms, he gradually developed an intermittent, itchy, commonly crusted, "allergic" rash above the elbows, buttocks, knees and above the shoulders. He was 18 when seen at the dermatology department with classical DH (Fig. 15.2), which was confirmed by skin histology and immunofluorescence. At that time his endomysium antibody (EMA) was positive. Under strict GFD he slowly became free of skin symptoms. There was no CD in the family by serological screening at that time,

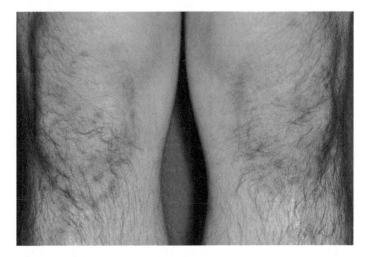

FIGURE 15.2 Typical crusted erosions above the knees

but anti-thyroid antibodies were identified in the patient without a functional endocrinological defect.

Key Points to Case 2

1. CD and DH are very closely related, as it is well illustrated with this case report. This case also demonstrates, that there are no genetic differences between the two diseases [4]. Severe CD is usually not associated with DH, mostly mild gluten induced enteropathy can induce the skin disease.
2. Associated other autoimmunities such as autoimmune thyroiditis, vitiligo, autoimmune diabetes mellitus or pernicious anemia are commonly associated with DH [3].
3. According to our current knowledge, strict GFD should be kept life-long.

Discussion

Dermatitis herpetiformis is unique within the group of autoimmune blistering diseases [1], because it is a gluten induced, reversible autoimmunity to transglutaminase 3 and 2 (TG3 and TG2) in the vast majority of the patients. Histologically it is characterized by granular IgA, complement 3 and TG 3 deposition in the perilesional papillary dermis, while within the skin symptoms also a subepidermal neutrophil accumulation and blister formation is present. Since neither the circulating IgA TG3 nor the IgA TG2 type autoantibodies bind along the dermal connective tissue of the normal papillary skin, the cutaneous disease is most probably of immune complex origin. DH is developing mainly among people with mild, latent form of CD and can be well treated by a life-long lasting, strict GFD. The time to complete skin remission, however, can last months, or longer. Under GF diet both the IgA type TG2 and TG3 autoantibodies gradually disappear from the circulation. CD and DH patients have a common genetic predisposition, best characterized by the HLA DQ2 (95 %) or HLADQ8 (5 %) haplotypes [4].

References

1. Kárpáti S. An exception within the group of autoimmune blistering diseases: dermatitis herpetiformis, the gluten sensitive dermopathy. Dermatol Clin. 2011;29:463–8.
2. Kárpáti S, Kósnai I, Török E, Kovács JB. Immunoglobulin A deposition in jejunal mucosa of children with dermatitis herpetiformis. J Invest Dermatol. 1988;91:336–9.
3. Reunala T, Collin P. Diseases associated with dermatitis herpetiformis. Br J Dermatol. 1997;136:315–8.
4. Spurkland A, Ingvarsson G, Falk ES, Knutsen I, Sollid LM, Thorsby E. Dermatitis herpetiformis and celiac disease are both primarily associated with the HLA-DQ (alpha 1*0501, beta 1*02) or the HLA-DQ (alpha 1*03, beta 1*0302) heterodimers. Tissue Antigens. 1997;49:29–34.

Chapter 16
A Healthy African Child with Blisters

Nokubonga F. Khoza and Anisa Mosam

A 3 year old child presented with a history of blisters for a period of 6 months. She had been treated at her local clinic for impetigo with repeated courses of antibiotics. The mum reported that the blisters would appear in crops, ulcerate, heal and a few weeks alter the cycle would repeat itself. There was no drug history, other than antibiotics and topical mupirocin for the lesions.

On examination, she had blisters and ulcers involving the groin, limbs and trunk. The blisters were tense and situated on the periphery of the ulcerated areas, progressing outward. The erosions were deep, revealing underlying dermis and there was no evidence of secondary infection. The blisters healed with a haemorrhagic scab.

Picture of scattered tense blisters with blistering progressing peripheral to the ulcerated area (Fig. 16.1).

What is the diagnosis?

1. Bullous Impetigo
2. Bullous insect bites

N.F. Khoza, MBChB, FC Derm
A. Mosam, MBChB, FC Derm, MMed (✉)
Department of Dermatology, Nelson R Mandela School of Medicine, University of Kwazulu-Natal, Durban, South Africa
e-mail: nokumas@yahoo.com

D.F. Murrell (ed.), *Clinical Cases in Autoimmune Blistering Diseases*, Clinical Cases in Dermatology 5, DOI 10.1007/978-3-319-10148-4_16,
© Springer International Publishing Switzerland 2015

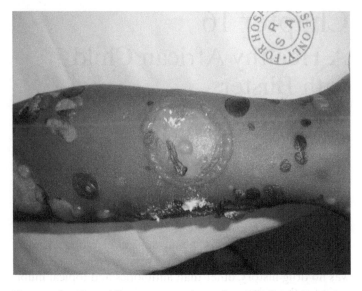

FIGURE 16.1 Tense blisters scattered over lower limb

3. Chronic Bullous disease of Childhood (CBDC)
4. Childhood bullous pemphigoid
5. Erythema multiforme

Subsequently Biopsy and IMF were performed. Biopsy revealed a subepidermal blister with a neutrophil rich infiltrate and IMF showed linear deposits of IgA at the DEJ.

The child was diagnosed as CBDC and therapy with Dapsone started at 2 mg/kg. A Blood count was done to check the haemoglobin prior to initiating therapy and Glucose-6-phosphate-dehydrogenase deficiency was excluded. Over the next few months on Dapsone, lesions healed and fewer blisters erupted. After 6 months of therapy, no new lesions occurred and the patient's Dapsone was stopped.

Chronic Bullous Disease of Childhood

Chronic bullous disease of childhood (CBDC) is an autoimmune blistering disease seen in children. It is self limiting in its course. It begins at least by age 2–3 years with average age of onset is 5 years. CBDC is a childhood variant of linear IgA disease, where circulating IgA autoantibodies against the basement membrane are the cause [1–2]. The immunoreactions IgA antibodies are found in three areas within the basement membrane zone, i.e. the lamina Lucida, at and below the lamina Lucida and above and below the lamina Lucida and therefore multiple targets against BP 230, BP180, and Type VII collagens [1–2].

The children present with tense blisters on an erythematous base or normal skin, these blisters are arranged in rosettes or an annular array forming a collarete of blisters, a clinical sign commonly referred to as the 'cluster of jewels'/ string of pearls [1–2]. Lesions typically affect the lower trunk, perineum (buttocks and genitalia), perioral and scalp lesions are also very common. The disease is diagnosed on skin biopsy of affected area by the identification of a sub epidermal blister that is neutrophil rich, neutrophils are along the basement membrane often accumulating in the papillary tips. Direct immunofluorescence test shows linear IgA deposits at the dermoepidermal junction [1–2]. The treatment of choice is dapsone however untreated; the disease runs a variable course, with spontaneous resolution by adolescence age [1–4].

Childhood Bullous Pemphigoid is also an autoimmune disease; it is rare, seen frequently less than 1 year of age and last for short duration 5 months or less. It is characterised by tense blisters on erythematous or urticated skin. The blisters are usually localised, acral in distribution beginning with bullae in the hands or feet and clinically blisters are not clustered. Histology in these patients shows IgG and C3 at the basement membrane zone and the blisters are predominantly eosinophilic rich. The antibodies are directed against hemidesmosomal proteins, BP 230 and BP180 [1, 5].

Bullous Impetigo is common in children at any age. Children present with bullae anywhere in the body commonly face, neck and hands, scalp is not involved. These patients may have pustular lesions as well. The bullae are large, fragile, crusted or weepy and leave circinate configuration when they rupture. The children may or may not experience constitutional symptoms. Lesions can spontaneously resolve or respond to oral and topical antibodies.

Erythema multiforme lesions can blister. The primary lesion is targetoid and blistering is usual at the centre of the lesion, the blisters are haemorrhagic with peripheral erythema and then hypopigmentation. Histology Bullous erythema multiforme is characterized by vacuolation at interface dermis and epidermis. The epidermis shows cellular necrosis which can be focal or confluent.

Epidermolysis Bullosa Congenita is a genetic disorder seen in children from birth or early childhood characterised by blisters at sites of injury or friction. There is usually a family history in these babies.

Children present with blisters from birth or soon after with tense or firm blisters at sites of friction. Common sites include trunk/flacks, buttock, occipital area, elbows and knees. Nail and mucosal involvement may occur. Healing in these patient is with hyperpigmentation and scarring.

References

1. Sansarica F, Stein SL, Petroni-Rosic V. Autoimmune bullous diseases in childhood. Clin Dermatol. 2012;30(1):114–27.
2. Mintz EM, Morel KD. Clinical features and pathogenesis of chronic bullous disease of childhood. Dermatol Clin. 2011;29(3): 459–62.
3. Mintz EM, Morel KD. Treatment of chronic bullous disease of childhood. Dermatol Clin. 2011;29(4):699–700.
4. Rados J. Autoimmune blistering diseases: histologic meaning. Clin Dermatol. 2011;29(4):377–88.
5. Aboobaker J, Wojnarowsa FT. Chronic bullous disease of childhood– clinical and immunological features seen in African patients. Clin Exp Dermatol. 1991;16(3):160–4.

Chapter 17
Case Report: An 11 Year-Old Girl with Blisters

Monia Kharfi

An 11-year-old Tunisian girl without any previous medical problems had a 1 month history of flaccid bullous lesions and large crusted hyperkeratotic erosions on the trunk, limbs, and face without mucosal involvement. There was no family history of autoimmune disease. No improvement was noted with a full course of systemic antibiotic treatment see Fig. 17.1.

A lesional biopsy was performed for histological analysis see Fig. 17.2.

Based on the case description, the clinical and histopathological pictures, what is your diagnosis?

1. Stevens-Johnson syndrome
2. IgA linear dermatosis
3. Pemphigus
4. Dermatitis herpetiformis
5. Epidermolysis bullosa

M. Kharfi, M.D., Ph.D.
Department of Dermatology,
Hôpital Charles Nicolle,
Tunis, Tunisia
e-mail: monia.kharfi@yahoo.fr

D.F. Murrell (ed.), *Clinical Cases in Autoimmune Blistering Diseases*, Clinical Cases in Dermatology 5, DOI 10.1007/978-3-319-10148-4_17,
© Springer International Publishing Switzerland 2015

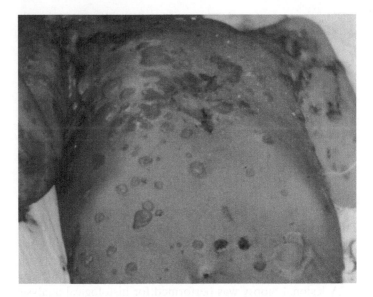

FIGURE 17.1 Clinical presentation

Diagnosis

Pemphigus foliaceus

Discussion

Pemphigus is an uncommon mucocutaneous disease caused by autoantibodies against desmosomal antigens. Juvenile cases are rare. The diagnosis is often delayed due to confusion with other entities.

The biopsy performed for our patient showed suprabasal acantholysis. Direct immunofluorescence (DIF) studies of frozen skin tissue showed positive intercellular staining for IgG within the epidermis. Blood samples for indirect immunofluorescence (IIF) on rabbit's esophagus demonstrated circulating IgG autoantibodies at a titer of 1:100.

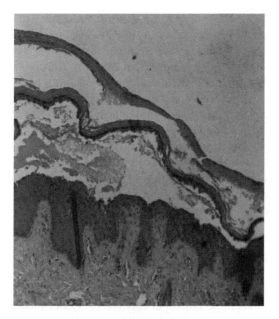

FIGURE 17.2 Histological presentation

A diagnosis of juvenile pemphigus vulgaris (PV) was made. Treatment was started with 1 mg/kg/d (50 mg/d) methylprednisolone. A gradual remission was observed. Complete regression of the lesion was obtained after 30 days, and the dose of methylprednisolone was gradually reduced after 45 days without any recurrence. No side effects were observed.

After 3 years the maintenance 5 mg/d methylprednisolone treatment was discontinued, and the girl has had no relapses over the last 7 years.

Pemphigus is a group of autoimmune blistering skin disease characterized by blister formation. Blisters are due to the loss of keratinocyte cell-cell adhesion in the superficial and deep epidermis [1].

Juvenile pemphigus is rare – except for the endemic form. Only 33 pediatric cases of PV [2] and 19 cases of PF have been reported.

Stomatitis is the presenting sign in more than 50 % of children with PV. In some cases, skin blisters may be the single symptom of PV, and no mucous membrane lesions are present.

PF is less frequent than PV in children. It presents as disseminated superficial flaccid bullous and erythematous lesions covered with seborrheic scabs [3].

The incidence rate of pemphigus in Tunisia is 6.7 cases per million per year. High rates of pemphigus foliaceus (PF) among young people living in rural areas are reminiscent of Brazilian pemphigus. However, the absence of cases among genetically related household members and during childhood, as well as the large predominance among women, contrasts with Brazilian pemphigus [4].

Differentials

In childhood, pemphigus may be misdiagnosed and confused with bullous impetigo, especially for PF. Other blistering diseases are more common in children such as dermatitis herpetiformis, IgA linear dermatosis, epidermolysis bullosa, and Stevens Johnson Syndrome. It requires a high index of suspicion in order to make an early diagnosis and to avoid treatment delay.

Treatment

Systemic corticosteroids are the treatment of choice for pemphigus vulgaris. Immunosuppressive agent (azathioprine, cyclophosphamide) could be added for patients with severe disease that cannot be controlled by corticosteroids alone or to reduce the dose of corticosteroids [2]. Children are extremely vulnerable to the side effects of systemic corticosteroids, notably infections and growth retardation. A successful use of rituximab therapy has been reported in refractory childhood pemphigus vulgaris [5]. Some authors recommend the use of intravenous immunoglobulins for cases of childhood and juvenile pemphigus, in which this therapy can delay the need for administration of immunosuppressive drugs [2].

Prognosis

Prognosis of pemphigus is usually better in childhood than in adulthood, except for paraneoplastic pemphigus (with little data on children). But PV also seems to show a relapsing course in the pediatric age group like in adults. However, as seen in our case, complete recovery is also possible.

In Conclusion

Pemphigus rarely occurs in childhood, but should be included in the differential diagnosis, particularly when a pediatric patient presents with chronic blisters.

References

1. Meyera N, Misery L. Geoepidemiologic considerations of auto-immune pemphigus. Autoimmun Rev. 2010;9(5):A379–82.
2. Mabrouk D, Ahmed AR. Analysis of current therapy and clinical outcome in childhood pemphigus vulgaris. Pediatr Dermatol. 2011;28(5):485–93.
3. Galambrun C, Cambazard F, Clavel C, et al. Pemphigus foliaceus. Arch Dis Child. 1997;77(3):255–7.
4. Zaraa I, Kerkeni N, Ishak F, et al. Spectrum of autoimmune blistering dermatoses in Tunisia. An 11-year study and review of the literature. Int J Dermatol. 2011;50(8):939–44.
5. Kanwar AJ, Sawatkar GU, Vinay K, Hashimoto T. Childhood pemphigus vulgaris successfully treated with rituximab. Indian J Dermatol Venereol Leprol. 2012;78(5):632–4.

Chapter 18
A Man with a Blistering Rash

Adam G. Harris and Dédée F. Murrell

A 31 year old caucasian male presented to his GP with a new onset erythematous and pruritic blistering rash to his groin and scalp.

He was treated with a topical antifungal and a potent topical steroid cream with no improvement.

He was referred to a dermatologist and by this time he had developed erythematous and pruritic blisters on his palms, arms, soles, penis, perianal area and in his mouth (see Fig. 18.1). He also complained of fragile skin, which lifted and blistered when it was rubbed. He had no personal or family history of blistering skin conditions, no significant past medical history and did not take any medications.

A.G. Harris, MBChB
Department of Dermatology, St George Hospital,
Level 0, James Laws House, St George Hospital, Gray Street,
Kogarah, Sydney, NSW 2217, Australia

D.F. Murrell, M.A., BMBCh, FAAD, M.D., FACD (✉)
Department of Dermatology, St George Hospital,
Level 0, James Laws House, St George Hospital, Gray Street,
Kogarah, Sydney, NSW 2217, Australia

University of New South Wales, Sydney, NSW Australia
e-mail: d.murrell@unsw.edu.au

D.F. Murrell (ed.), *Clinical Cases in Autoimmune Blistering Diseases*, Clinical Cases in Dermatology 5, DOI 10.1007/978-3-319-10148-4_18, © Springer International Publishing Switzerland 2015

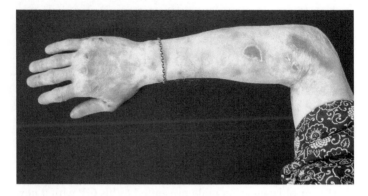

FIGURE 18.1 A man with a blistering rash

A skin biopsy was taken which showed a subepidermal blister with neutrophils and occasional eosinophils. PAS staining showed that the basement membrane was in the floor of the blister. Immunohistochemistry showed C3 was deposited along the dermoepidermal junction and around the appendages and fibrinogen in the floor of the blister.

He was commenced on Prednisone 60 mg daily, but despite this, new blisters continued to develop. These occurred generally around sites of trauma and old blisters healed with scarring and milia.

Based on the case description and photographs, what is your preferred diagnosis?

1. Dystrophic Epidermolysis Bullosa
2. Epidermolysis Bullosa Acquisita
3. Bullous Pemphigoid
4. Bullous Systemic Lupus Erythematosus

His prednisone dose was increased to a maximum of 280 mg a day and trials of Dapsone 200 mg daily, Tetracycline 1.5 gm daily, Doxycycline 200 mg daily and Azathioprine at

200 mg daily were used with little improvement in an attempt to control the disease.

A repeated skin biopsy showed a subepidermal blister with lymphocytic and eosinophilic inflammation and positive IgG and C3 along the split on direct immunofluorescence (IF). Indirect IF on human salt-split skin was positive in a strong linear band at the floor of the split. Serum for Western immunoblot testing confirmed autoantibodies to type VII collagen.

Blistering continued despite trials of Colchicine, Cyclosporin A, intravenous immunoglobulin, photophoresis, Sulfasalazine, Mycophenylate and Methotrexate. He developed progressive dysphagia due to esophageal strictures, which resulted in profound weight loss and nutritional deficiencies [1].

The decision was made to trial Rituximab, which was given in four infusions over 3 months at a dose of 375 mg per meter squared of body surface area.

Within 2 months of having the first dose of Rituximab, the amount of new blistering lesions dramatically diminished and he was weaned off Prednisone. Four months after the first infusion, his dysphagia had markedly improved and with an increased oral intake he gained 12 kg in weight (see Fig. 18.2a Pre-Rituximab and 2B Post-Rituximab).

Diagnosis

Epidermolysis Bullosa Acquisita

Discussion

Epidermolysis Bullosa Acquistia (EBA) is a rare, acquired and chronic autoimmune blistering disease characterized by IgG autoantibodies against type VII collagen resulting in

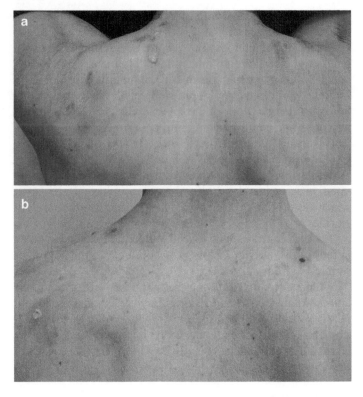

FIGURE 18.2 (a) EBA pre-Rituximab, (b) EBA post-Rituximab

subepidermal blistering with minimal trauma to the skin [2]. EBA presents with generalized blistering and subsequent erosions with associated pruritus, erythema, skin fragility (positive Nikolsky's sign) and healing with scarring and formation of milia. Type VII collagen is a major component of the anchoring fibrils in the basement membrane zone, which help maintain the adhesion of the dermis to the epidermis. It is the same protein that is affected in hereditary Dystrophic Epidermolysis Bullosa (DEB), which EBA resembles clinically and from which EBA originally derived its name.

DEB is a genetic condition with a defect in the CO7A1 gene that codes for type VII collagen [3]. The recessive and most severe form of DEB usually presents early on in life and is associated with premature mortality [4]. Treatment consists of protective and therapeutic dressings, use of topical preparations and prevention and treatment of complications of the disease. Translational therapies, including gene, cell and protein therapies are in the development phases [5].

EBA can also be clinically indistinguishable from Bullous Pemphigoid (BP), which is the most common autoimmune blistering disease in the older generation. BP is characterized by autoantibodies against the BP180 and BP 230 antigens, which are components of the hemidesmosome adhesion complex [6]. BP normally presents with spontaneous tense blistering, intense pruritus and is not usually associated with skin fragility (negative Nikolsky's sign), trauma induced blisters, scarring or milia. Histologically BP is similar to EBA with subepidermal blistering and a linear deposit of IgG and C3 at the BMZ. Indirect IF is most commonly used on salt-split-skin to differentiate the two conditions, where autoantibodies are detected on the dermal side of the split in EBA and on the epidermal or both sides in BP. If differentiation is still unclear, Western immunoblot testing, immunoelectron microscopy (IEM) or type VII collagen ELISA (enzyme linked immunoassay studies) can be performed [7]. BP tends to be more responsive to corticosteroid treatment whereas EBA tends to be resistant. EBA has been shown to respond to Dapsone, Cyclosporin A, Mycophenylate, photophoresis and Rituximab [8].

Blistering occurs in 5 % of cases of Systemic Lupus Erythematous with a subgroup of these being categorized as Bullous Systemic Lupus Erythematous (BSLE). This disease is believed to be caused by autoantibodies to type VII collagen, similar to that affected EBA and DEB [9]. BSLE typically occurs as an acute eruption with no skin fragility (negative Nilkosky's sign), minimal pruritus and does not heal with scarring or millia, unlike EBA. BSLE generally responds very well to Dapsone and there has been some success with immunosuppressive therapies [9].

Based on the clinical history and the positive Western immunoblot test to type VII collagen, a diagnosis of EBA in this case was made. Interestingly, he was resistant to most immunosuppressive therapies but showed a dramatic improvement with Rituximab. Rituximab is a monoclonal antibody, which targets CD20 positive B lymphocytes resulting in their depletion in the circulation [10]. In EBA, this is thought to result in a reduced amount of pathogenic antibodies directed at the BMZ [11]. Rituximab is widely used in other autoimmune conditions, including Pemphigus Vulgaris [12] and has been shown to be successful in other cases of recalcitrant EBA [11].

Key Points

- Bullous Pemphigoid is the most common autoimmune bullous disease of the elderly.
- When BP is suspected, EBA should be considered as a differential diagnosis, especially so if there is a history of trauma induced blisters, fragile skin, healing with scarring or milia and resistance to treatment with high dose corticosteroids.
- EBA is diagnosed by a combination of clinical history and indirect IF on salt-split-skin, Western immunoblot testing, immunoelectron microscopy or ELISA.
- Rituximab is a novel new treatment for EBA.
- EBA, BP, DEB and BSLE are all differential diagnoses for a blistering rash, see Table 18.1 for a summary of distinguishing features of each.

TABLE 18.1 Comparative characteristics of EBA, RDEB, BP and BSLE [2]

	EBA	BP	RDEB	BSLE
Age of onset	Adults and children	Elderly	Birth, childhood	Adults
Etiology	Autoimmune	Autoimmune	Genetic	Autoimmune
Pattern on direct immunofluorescence	Linear BMZ	Linear BMZ	N/A	Linear BMZ
Location of antibodies on saltsplit-skin	Dermal	Epidermal or mixed (epidermal and dermal)	N/A	Dermal
Affected protein	Type VII collagen	BP230, BP180	Type VII collagen	Type VII collagen
Distribution	Generalized, variable, sites of trauma	Trunks, limbs, flexures	Generalized, sites of trauma	Generalized, variable
Healing	Scarring and milia	No scarring, no milia	Scarring and milia	No scarring, no milia
Nikolsky's sign	Positive	Negative	Positive	Negative
Treatment	Corticosteroids, dapsone, immunosuppressive therapy	Corticosteroids, dapsone, immunosuppressive therapy	Prevention and treatment of complications, experimental therapies	Dapsone

References

1. Shipman AR, Agero AL, Scolyer RA, Craig P, Pas HH, Wonjnarowska F, Murrell DF. Epidermolysis bullosa acquisita requiring multiple oesophageal dilatations. Clin Exp Dermatol. 2008;33:776–94.
2. Burns T, Breathnach S, Cox N, Griffiths C. Rook's dermatology. 8th ed; 2010. Pages section 40.51–40.56.
3. Dang N, Murrell DF. Mutation analysis and characterization of COL7A1 mutations in dystrophic epidermolysis bullosa. Exp Dermatol. 2008;17:553–68.
4. Fine JD, Johnson LB, Weiner M, Suchindran C. Cause specific risks of childhood death in inherited epidermolysis bullosa. J Pediatr. 2008;152(2).
5. Venugopal SS, Yan W, Frew JW, Cohn HI, Rhodes LM, Tran K, Melbourne W, Nelson JA, Sturm A, Fogarty J, Marinkovich PM, Igawa S, Ishida-Yamamoto A, Murrell DF. A phase II randomized vehicle-controlled trial of intradermal allogeneic fibroblasts for recessive dystrophic epidermolysis bullosa. J Am Acad Dermatol. 2014;69(6):899.
6. Gammon WA, Brigaman RA, Woodley DT, Heald PW, Wheller CE. Epidermolysis bullosa acquisita a Pemphigoid-like disease. J Am Acad Dermatol. 1984;11:5, Part 1, Nov 1984.
7. Chan YC, Sun YJ, Ng PL, Tan SH. Comparison of immunofluorescence microscopy, immunoblotting and enzyme-linked immunosorbent assay methods in the laboratory diagnosis of bullous Pemphigoid. Clin Exp Dermatol. 2003;28:651–6.
8. Intong LR, Murrell DF. Management of epidermolysis bullosa acquisita. Dermatol Clin. 2011;29(2011):643–7.
9. Sebaratnam DF, Murrell DF. Bullous systemic lupus erythematosus. Dermatol Clin. 2011;29(2011):649–53. doi:10.1016/j.det.2011.06.002.
10. Cerny T, Borisch B, Introna M, Johnson P, Rose AL. Mechanism of action of rituximab. Anticancer Drugs. 2002;13 suppl 2:S3–10.
11. Kim JH, Lee SE, Kim S. Successful treatment of epidermolysis bullosa acquisita with rituximab therapy. J Dermatol. 2011;477.
12. Diaz L. Rituximab and Pemphigus – a therapeutic advance. N Engl J Med. 2007; 357:6.

Chapter 19
A Chronically Ill Teenager with Blisters and Scars

Nokubonga F. Khoza and Anisa Mosam

A 15 year old patient presented with a 6 month history of painful blisters. She was chronically unwell and complained of loss of weight, malaise, alopecia and oral ulcers. On examination the blisters were scattered on the trunk, limbs and there was evidence of scarring from previous blisters. The blisters were on a non-inflammatory base, some were haemorrhagic and there was evidence of atrophy and secondary leucoderma.

Figure 19.1 showing varying sizes of bullae on the limb.

Figure 19.2 demonstrating an active blister with the background of an ulcer and secondary leucoderma

What is your diagnosis?

EBA
Bullous Pemphigoid
Cicatricial Pemphigoid
Bullous SLE

N.F. Khoza, MBChB, FC Derm
A. Mosam, MBChB, FC Derm, MMed, Ph.D. (✉)
Department of Dermatology, Nelson R Mandela School of Medicine,
University of Kwazulu-Natal, Durban, South Africa
e-mail: nokumas@yahoo.com

D.F. Murrell (ed.), *Clinical Cases in Autoimmune Blistering Diseases*, Clinical Cases in Dermatology 5, DOI 10.1007/978-3-319-10148-4_19,
© Springer International Publishing Switzerland 2015

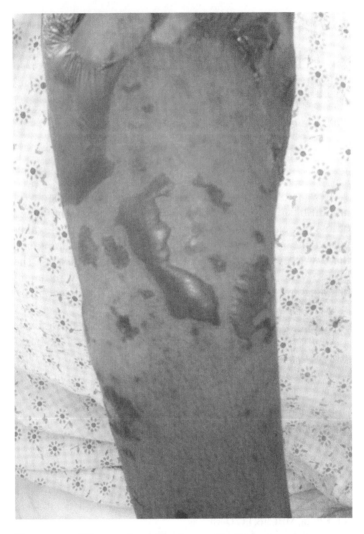

FIGURE 19.1 Blisters of varying sizes on the limb

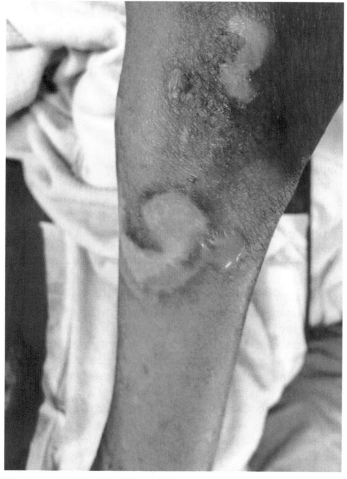

FIGURE 19.2 An active blister with the background of an ulcer and secondary leucoderma

Biopsy showed a subepidermal blister with cell poor infiltrate and IFM was positive for IgG, C3 and IgM at the DEJ. She was found to have low complement C3 and ANF was positive in a titre of 1: 1250.

This patient was diagnosed with Bullous SLE and therapy with prednisone started at 0.5 mg/kg and Dapsone.

Bullous SLE

Bullous LE is an autoimmune blistering condition, often transient that occurs in the setting of systemic lupus erythematosus. It is commonly seen in young female patients of African descent [1–2].

Bullous lesions of Lupus Erythematosus can be single or widespread. They are commonly but not limited to sun exposed areas [1–2]. These lesions are painful but not pruritic. Patients with bullous lupus erythematosus meet the criteria for systemic lupus erythematosus hence (bullous SLE), but patient do exist with similar lesions but have fewer symptoms to meet the criteria (disease in evolution [1]). The occurrence of blisters is not related to flares of systemic disease [1]. Histology shows a sub-epidermal blister rich in neutrophils. Direct Immunofluorescence shows IgG, IgA, IgM and C3 in a granular or linear pattern at the basement membrane zone [1]. These antibodies target type VII collagen. Dapsone is first line therapy and is most effective [1–2].

Epidermolysis Bullousa Acquisita is a mechano-bullous disease that share similar antibodies to bullous sle against basement membrane is characterised by skin fragility, the skin lesions have a predilection for traumatized areas, dorsa of the hands, elbows and fee. These heal with scarring and milia and hyperpigmentation [2–4].

Cicatricial pemphigoid commonly occurs in older women. Patient present with vesicles and blisters that rupture quickly. These primarily occur in mucous membranes, of the conjunctiva and oral mucosa. They are very severe and lead to scarring. Cutaneous lesions seen in 25 % of the patients, and distribution is any area. Histology is similar to bullous pemphigoid however there may be noticeable fibrosis and scarring in the upper dermis [2, 4].

Bullous Pemphigoid is also an autoimmune disease characterised by tense blisters on urticarial or erythematous base. Histology in these patients shows IgG and C3 at the basement membrane zone and the blisters are predominantly eosinophilic rich. The antibodies are directed against hemidesmosomal proteins, BP 230 and BP180 [2, 4].

References

1. Sebaratnam DF, Murrel DF: Bullous systemic erythematosus. Dermatol Clin. 2011;29(3):649–53k.
2. Sansarica Freda, Stein SL, Petroni-Rosic Vesna: Autoimmune bullous diseases in childhood. Clin Dermatol. 2012;30(1):114–27.
3. Lizbeth R.A Intong, Murrel DF. Management of Epidermolysis Bullosa Acquisita. Dermatol Clin. 2011;29(4):643–47.
4. Rados J. Autoimmune blistering diseases: histologic meaning. Clin Dermatol. 2011;29(4):377–88.

Chapter 20
Detached Epidermis in an Adult Female

Nayera H. Moftah

A 30-year-old female was referred to Al-Zahra University Hospital, Egypt, and presented with a generalized skin rash associated with fever, photophobia, blurring of vision and difficulty swallowing of sudden onset and progressive course. The skin lesions were composed of dusky erythematous macules with flaccid hemorrhagic bullae and areas of epidermal detachment. The lesions were generalized, involving the face, neck, trunk, both upper and lower limbs, with hands and feet, affecting about 60 % of body surface area Mucous membrane lesions were in the form of hemorrhagic crusts and erosions on the lips, erosions of the buccal mucosa and eye involvement (Fig. 20.1).

The condition was preceded by high grade fever 5 days earlier along with upper respiratory tract infection and epigastric pain for which she was prescribed co-trimoxazole (Septrin®), diclofenac sodium (Voltaren®), ranitidine tablets (Zantac®) for 4 days. She noticed no improvement and consulted another doctor, who shifted her to azithromycin tablets (Zithromax®) and ibuprofen tablets (Brufen®). The following day the patient developed the present condition.

N.H. Moftah, M.D.
Department of Dermatology and Venereology,
Faculty of Medicine for Girls, Al-Azhar University, Cairo, Egypt
e-mail: nayeramoftah@hotmail.com

D.F. Murrell (ed.), *Clinical Cases in Autoimmune*   143
Blistering Diseases, Clinical Cases in Dermatology 5,
DOI 10.1007/978-3-319-10148-4_20,
© Springer International Publishing Switzerland 2015

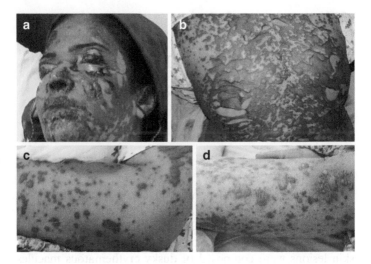

Figure 20.1 (a) Epidermal sloughing on face with affection of the eyes and lips. (b) Epidermal sloughing on the back. (c, d) Hemorrhagic flaccid blisters on upper and lower limbs

1. What is your diagnosis?

   (a) DRESS
   (b) Stevens Johnson syndrome
   (c) Toxic epidermal necrolysis
   (d) Erythroderma
   (e) Acute generalized exanthematous pustulosis

2. The drug associated with confirmed high risk of this skin disease is:

   (a) Ibuprofen
   (b) Co-trimoxazole
   (c) Diclofenac sodium
   (d) Azithromycin
   (e) Ranitidine

The patient was hospitalized in the intensive care unit where blood pressure was 110/70, pulse 90 /min with normal rhythm and temperature was 39 °C. CBC was normal, ESR is high (100 mm/min), elevated SGOT, SGPT (less than triple the normal values), low level of potassium (2.8 mmol/L), elevated level of urea and creatinine (113 mg/dL, 2.3 mg/dL) and normal glucose (post prandial: 135 mg/dL) and bicarbonate levels (22 mEq/L). All medications were stopped. Supportive treatment was given, fluid and electrolytes were corrected. Urea and creatinine became normal in 24 h. Then, Cyclosporine 5 mg/kg was started in addition to plasmapheresis which was done every other day for 2 weeks. Three weeks later, there were significant healing of eroded skin all over the body while oral lesions showed little improvement and symblepharon developed in the eyes (Fig. 20.2).

Diagnosis: Toxic epidermal necrolysis (Lyell's disease).

Answers

1. (c)
2. (b)

Discussion

Toxic epidermal necrolysis (TEN) is a life threatening adverse drug reaction (mortality rate 30 %) involving widespread keratinocyte apoptosis. TEN is characterized by

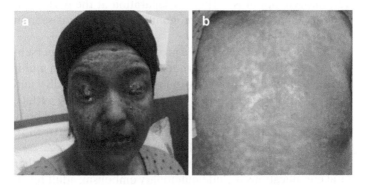

FIGURE 20.2 Improvement of skin lesions after 3 weeks

widespread sloughing of the skin and the mucosa. Drug-induced CD8 cell activation is highly specific for particular HLA allotypes, placing certain populations at a greater risk for developing TEN [1].

The majority of cases of toxic epidermal necrosis are the result of a hypersensitivity reaction to a drug. Other causative agents include Mycoplasma pneumonia, dengue virus, cytomegalovirus, and contrast medium [1]. According to the 2008 Euro-SCAR study [2], drugs associated with confirmed high risk of SJS/TEN includes nevirapine, lamotrigine, carbamazepine, phenytoin, phenobarbital, cotrimoxazole, other anti-infective sulphonamides, sulphasalazine, allopurinol, oxicam-non steroidal anti-inflammatory drugs;

TEN most often begin with a prodrome of fever, malaise, anorexia, pharyngitis, headache, and rash, A painful macular exanthem appears in a symmetrical distribution on the face and trunk, spreading to the extremities. The skin develops the Nikolsky sign, whereby gentle lateral pressure causes the epidermis to slide over the basal layer. Blisters evolve and large sheets of epidermis slough off, leaving an exposed, weeping dermis. Ocular involvement with adhesions and ulceration can result in photophobia, pain, and loss of vision. TEN is more commonly seen with HIV, systemic lupus erythematosus collagen vascular diseases and malignancy [3]. Histologically, sections of skin from TEN exhibit widespread keratinocyte apoptosis. There is separation at the dermoepidermal junction and a mild mononuclear infiltrate is seen in the dermis [4].

TEN is considered part of a group of cutaneous hypersensitivity reactions with a spectrum of severity; erythema multiforme, followed by Stevens-Johnson syndrome (SJS) and TEN. SJS involves less than 10 % of the total body surface area, whereas TEN involves more than 30 % of the total body surface area. Total body surface area involvement between 10 and 30 % is known as SJS-TEN overlap [5].

Infection is the most common cause of death in TEN. Other fatal complications include pulmonary embolism, adult respiratory distress syndrome, gastrointestinal hemorrhage, as well as cardiac and renal failure [6].

Distinguishing TEN syndrome from the other major potentially life-threatening cutaneous drug reactions with similar clinical features—Drug reactions with eosinophilia and systemic symptoms (DRESS), acute generalized exanthematous pustulosis (AGEP), and erythroderma (exfoliative dermatitis)—is an important concern because treatment varies among these conditions. Clinically, the onset of eruption of SJS/TEN, AGEP, and erythroderma after drug ingestion is shorter and subsides sooner than in DRESS syndrome. DRESS syndrome is characterized by facial edema, morbilliform eruption, pustules, exfoliative dermatitis, tense bullae, and possible target lesions. Lymph node enlargement, hepatitis and eosinophilia are also found [7].

AGEP is first evident as an edematous erythema in the body folds and face before generalizing to widespread non-follicular sterile pustules. It is associated with fever and neutrophilia, and spontaneously resolves in a few days. Like TEN and DRESS syndrome, it may result from a medication, often antibiotics or anticonvulsants, although it may be caused by a viral infection [8].

Erythroderma, also referred to as generalized exfoliative dermatitis, is characterized by erythema and scaling of 90 % of the body surface area. It is classified as being caused by one of four etiologies: a flare of a preexisting skin disorder, such as psoriasis or atopic dermatitis; a drug eruption; a lymphoma/leukemia, such as mycosis fungoides; or idiopathic. Allopurinol is one of the most common causes of drug-induced erythroderma [9].

Treatment of TEN: Patients have to be admitted to intensive care or special burns units if they have significant skin necrosis and detachment. If the patient is conscious and able to sit/stand he can be treated in the high dependency unit (HDU). The cornerstone of TEN treatment is early cessation of the causative drug, meticulous skin care, fluid management, nutritional support, and surveillance as well as treatment of infections. General supportive measures include increasing the room temperature to 30–32 °C to reduce caloric loss through the skin, and anticoagulation with subcutaneous heparin or low molecular weight heparin to prevent deep vein thrombosis in immobile patients for the duration of their hospital stay. Pulmonary care is instituted via the use of aerosols, bronchial aspiration and physiotherapy [10].

Skin care: Regular fluid release from fresh bullae using sterile needles, leaving the epidermis intact as its own dressing [11]. Various biological dressings have also been suggested, as well as silver dressings due to their inherent antimicrobial properties. There are some reports of success with skin allotransplantation and hyperbaric oxygen [12]. Daniel et al. [11] advocated easy cleaning with a spray-on bacteriologically pure thermal spring water spray (ATSW, Avene, France) and non-stick silicone dressings to areas where the skin had sloughed. A well skin healing occurred without infection or scarring.

Eye care: It is especially important in TEN. It was found that those given ocular topical steroids at disease onset had a statistically significantly better visual outcome [13]. The use of preservative-free lubricant eyedrops is recommended as preservatives cause ocular surface damage. Furthermore, eyedrops containing non-steroidal anti-inflammatories are to be avoided due to iatrogenic effects in this group of patients [14].

Adjuvant medication controversy: No established standard or specific medical treatment for TEN. Neither Intravenous immunoglobulin (IVIG) nor corticosteroids had any significant effect on mortality in comparison with supportive care only, although a trend for a beneficial effect of corticosteroids was noted [15]. IVIG has been used as an off label treatment for TEN. A prospective, open study conducted in 34 patients given 2.0 g/kg of IVIG within 2 days showed no benefit in mortality or progression [16].

Mycophenolate mofetil, ciclosporin, plasmapheresis, thalidomide and dapsone have all been tried with varying success in small case series, and mostly in conjunction with corticosteroids [17, 10, 18].

Recently, HLA genotype testing, to prevent the administration of drugs to susceptible individuals, has proven to be an important tool in the prevention of TEN. However, These HLA studies are still limited and variable in the different ethnicities [1].

Key Features

1. Constitutional symptoms, flaccid bullae with epidermal detachment in >30 % of body surface area and positive Nikolsky sign are essential for diagnosis of TEN
2. Oral and ocular mucosa are affected in all patients.
3. Early intervention with supportive treatment and adjunctive medication is the key.
4. IVIG has yet to be proven to be of any greater benefit in TEN than corticosteroids and is much more expensive [19].

References

1. Schwartz RA, McDonough PH, Lee BW. Toxic epidermal necrolysis. Part I. Introduction, history, classification, clinical features, systemic manifestations, etiology, and immunopathogenesis. J Am Acad Dermatol. 2013;69:173.e1–13.
2. Mockenhaupt M, Viboud C, Dunant A, Naldi L, Halevy S, Bouwes Bavinck JN, et al. Stevens-Johnson syndrome and toxic epidermal necrolysis: assessment of medication risks with emphasis on recently marketed drugs. The EuroSCAR study. J Invest Dermatol. 2008;128:35–44.
3. Wolff K, Goldsmith LA, Katz SI, Gilchrest BA, Paller AS, Lefell DJ. Fitzpatrick's dermatology in general medicine. 7th ed. New York: McGraw Hill; 2007.
4. Quinn AM, Brown K, Bonish BK, Curry J, Gordon KB, Sinacore J, Gamelli R, Nickoloff BJ. Uncovering histologic criteria with prognostic significance in toxic epidermal necrolysis. Arch Dermatol. 2005;141:683–7.

5. Downey A, Jackson C, Harun N, Cooper A. Toxic epidermal necrolysis: review of pathogenesis and management. J Am Acad Dermatol. 2012;66:995–1003.

6. Mukasa Y, Craven N. Management of toxic epidermal necrolysis and related syndromes. Postgrad Med J. 2008;84:60–5.

7. Bocquet H, Bagot M, Roujeau JC. Drug-induced pseudolymphoma and drug hypersensitivity syndrome (drug rash with eosinophilia and systemic symptoms: DRESS). Semin Cutan Med Surg. 1996;15:250–7.

8. Guevara-Gutierrez E, Uribe-Jimenez E, Diaz-Canchola M, Tlacuilo- Parra A. Acute generalized exanthematous pustulosis: report of 12 cases and literature review. Int J Dermatol. 2009;48: 253–8.

9. Okoduwa C, Lambert WC, Schwartz RA, Kubeyinje E, Eitokpah A, Sinha S, et al. Erythroderma: review of a potentially life-threatening dermatosis. Indian J Dermatol. 2009;54:1–6.

10. Letko E, Papaliodis DN, Papaliodis GN, et al. Stevens–Johnson syndrome and toxic epidermal necrolysis: a review of literature. Ann Allergy Asthma Immunol. 2005;94:419–36.

11. Daniel BS, Skowronski G, Myburgh J, Hersch M, Murrell DF. Concurrent management of toxic epidermal necrolysis with thermal water spray and non-stick dressings. Acta Dermatovenerol Croat. 2012;20:203–20.

12. Abood GJ, Nickoloff BJ, Gamelli RL. Treatment strategies in toxic epidermal necrolysis syndrome: where are we at? J Burn Care Res. 2008;29:269–76.

13. Sotozono C, Ueta M, Koizumi N, et al. Diagnosis and treatment of Stevens–Johnson syndrome and toxic epidermal necrolysis with ocular complications. Ophthalmology. 2009;116:685–90.

14. Gueudry J, Roujeau JC, Binaghi M, et al. Risk factors for the development of ocular complications of Stevens–Johnson syndrome and toxic epidermal necrolysis. Arch Dermatol. 2009;145:157–62.

15. Schneck J, Fagot JP, Sekula P, et al. Effects of treatments on the mortality of Stevens–Johnson syndrome and toxic epidermal necrolysis: a retrospective study on patients included in the prospective EuroSCAR study. J Am Acad Dermatol. 2008;58: 33–40.

16. Bachot N, Revuz J, Roujeau JC. Intravenous immunoglobulin treatment for Stevens–Johnson syndrome and toxic epidermal necrolysis. Arch Dermatol. 2003;139:33–6.

17. Borchers AT, Lee JL, Naguwa SM, et al. Stevens–Johnson syndrome and toxic epidermal necrolysis. Autoimmun Rev. 2008;7:598–605.
18. Majumdar S, Mockenhaupt M, Roujeau JC, et al. Interventions for toxic epidermal necrolysis. Cochrane Database Syst Rev. 2002;4:CD001435.
19. Intong LRA, Murrell DF. Erythema multiforme, Stevens–Johnson syndrome and toxic epidermal necrolysis. In: Irvine A, Hoeger P and Yan A, editors. Textbook of pediatric dermatology, 3rd edition. Oxford: Blackwell Publishing Ltd. 2011.

Chapter 21
Single Step Multivariant Analysis of Serum Autoantibodies in Autoimmune Blistering Diseases Using BIOCHIP® Mosaic Technology

Nina van Beek and Enno Schmidt

Case 1: An Elderly Male with Chronic Pruritic Erythema

A 78-year-old Caucasian male has been referred with erythema on the lower back, buttocks and thighs. He complained of severe itching for several months. The accompanying nurse reported that the first skin lesions had appeared 3 months ago and since then constantly increased in size and numbers. The patient did not recognize any blisters and the nurse is not sure of having seen blisters. The patient also suffered from diabetes and dementia and was on several medications. On examination gyrated, urticaria-like erythema and erosions

N. van Beek • E. Schmidt, M.D., Ph.D. (✉)
Department of Dermatology, University of Luebeck,
Ratzeburger Allee 160, D-23538 Lübeck, Germany
e-mail: vanbeek@uksh.de; enno.schmidt@uksh.de

D.F. Murrell (ed.), *Clinical Cases in Autoimmune Blistering Diseases*, Clinical Cases in Dermatology 5, DOI 10.1007/978-3-319-10148-4_21,
© Springer International Publishing Switzerland 2015

153

were found on the lower back. A single tense blister was present on the right thigh.

Blood was taken for autoantibody analysis which was performed by indirect immunofluorescence (IF) microscopy using BIOCHIP™ technology (Fig. 21.1).

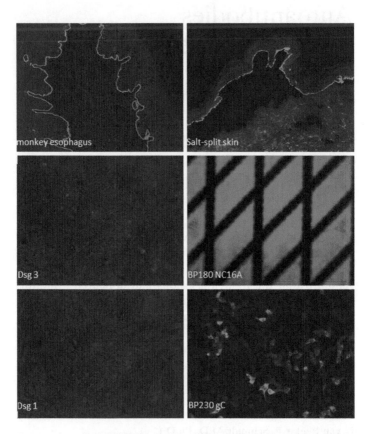

Figure 21.1 **BIOCHIP™ mosaic after incubation with a bullous pemphigoid serum**. Reactivity is seen with the dermal-epidermal junction of monkey esophagus and human salt-split skin as well as with recombinant BP180 NC16A directly coated on the BIOCHIP™ and BP230gC (C-terminal globular domain of BP230)-expressing HEK293 cells. No staining is observed with Desmoglein (Dsg) 1- and Dsg3-expressing HEK293 cells [9]

Which differential diagnosis can be made based on the BIOCHIP™ mosaic results and the case description?

1. Epidermolysis bullosa acquisita
2. Bullous pemphigoid
3. Anti-p200/laminin γ1 pemphigoid
4. Pemphigoid gestationis
5. Drug eruption

Diagnosis

Bullous Pemphigoid

Case 2: A 46-Year-Old Female with Oral Erosions

A 46-year-old female was referred by her dentist with a 9-months history of erosions on the gingiva and right buccal mucosa. The lesions have been worsening during the course of the disease and led to a weight loss of 5 kg due to painful food intake. On examination in addition to the oral lesions, haemorrhagic crusts were found on the nasal mucosa and two crusted erosions on the chest and upper abdomen. Conjunctivae and genitalia were not involved.

Further workup included serological testing for autoimmune bullous disorders by BIOCHIP™ technology (Fig. 21.2).

Based on the case report and the BIOCHIP™ mosaic result, what diagnosis can be made?

1. Pemphigus foliaceus
2. Staphylococcal scaled skin syndrome
3. Pemphigus vulgaris
4. Oral herpes infection
5. Mucous membrane pemphigoid

Diagnosis

Pemphigus Vulgaris

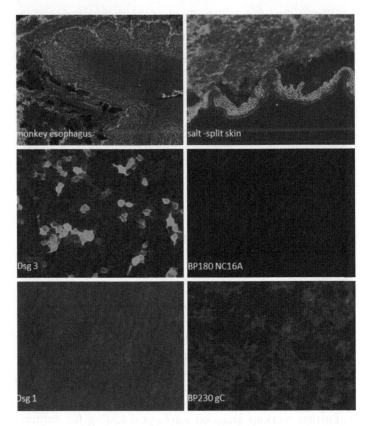

FIGURE 21.2 **BIOCHIP™ mosaic after incubation with a pemphigus vulgaris serum**. Intercellular labeling of the epithelium of monkey oesophagus and staining of Desmoglein (Dsg) 3-expressing HEK293 cells can be seen. No reactivity with the dermal-epidermal junction of salt-split human skin and the other substrates is observed [9]

Discussion

In the group of autoimmune bullous disorders, the identification of target antigens enables physicians to differentiate between these frequently clinically similar appearing bullous diseases. Advances in the discovery of new antigens and the subsequent development of an increasing number of sensitive and specific assays for the detection of circulating auto-antibodies allow the serological diagnosis in the majority of patients [1]. While the diagnostic gold standard is still the direct IF microscopy of a perilesional biopsy, in the majority of patients, diagnosis can be made by the combination of clinical findings and serology.

A step-wise analysis is usually employed starting with indirect IF microscopy using tissue sections (e.g. monkey esophagus for pemphigus and salt-split skin i.e. normal human skin in which the dermal-epidermal junction was separated by incubation in 1 M NaCl solution) followed by ELISA. At present, six ELISA systems based on the recombinant target antigens are available: desmoglein 1, desmoglein 3, BP180, BP230, type VII collagen, and envoplakin [2–8]. In some patients, additional analyses such as immunoblotting and immunoprecipitation are required to detect autoantibodies against e.g. laminin 332, the ectodomain of BP180, periplakin, and $\alpha 2$ macroglobulin-like 1. These assays are only available in specialized laboratories.

To facilitate the serological diagnosis of immunobullous disorders, a multiplex IF–based BIOCHIP™ mosaic has been developed that combines screening and target antigen-specific substrates in a single miniature incubation field. This novel assay contains HEK293 cells transfected with the membrane-bound extracellular domains of desmoglein 1 and desmoglein 3, the C-terminal globular domain of BP230 (BP230gC), recombinant tetrameric NC16A (BP180-NC16A-4X), and tissue sections of monkey esophagus and primate 1 M NaCl-split skin in a single incubation field of 5×5 mm. A FITC-conjugated IgG/IgA mixture is applied as detection antibody. Sensitivities and specificities of the BIOCHIP™ mosaic were comparable to those of the individual ELISA systems. Sensitivities of the desmoglein 1-, desmoglein 3-, and NC16A-specific substrates were 90 %, 98.5 % and 100 %. BP230 was recognized by 54 % of the bullous pemphigoid sera. Specificities ranged from 98.2 % to 100 % for all substrates [9].

In **Case 1**, the BIOCHIP™ mosaic diagnostics of the patient's serum showed both, linear reactivity at the dermal-epidermal junction on salt split skin and monkey esophagus as well as positive staining with the recombinant immuno-dominant domain of BP180. This patient thus suffers from a BP180-positive, BP230-negative bullous pemphigoid. The signs and symptoms he described are well compatible with the prodromal phase of the disease in which severe pruritus and erythematous, eczematous or urticarial skin lesions may be found [8]. The same IF pattern by BIOCHIP™ mosaic could be found in patients with pemphigoid gestationis, mucous membrane pemphigoid, and linear IgA dermatosis, the first two diseases would need to be differentiated clinically.

In **Case 2**, the BIOCHIP™ mosaic diagnostic revealed the diagnosis of pemphigus vulgaris since an IF staining was seen on monkey oesophagus in an intercellular pattern and with desmoglein 3-expressing cells. Paraneoplastic pemphigus may be excluded by e.g. indirect IF microscopy on rat-or monkey bladder and envoplakin ELISA. Alternatively, reactivity against envoplakin, periplakin, and desmoplakin can be determined by Western blotting or immunoprecipitation of extract of cultured keratinocytes; both tests are only available in specialized laboratories.

Comparing the routine multistep diagnostic procedure applied at the department of dermatology, University of Luebeck, Germany [10], with the BIOCHIP™ mosaic a high agreement was found between the results for the diagnosis of bullous pemphigoid, pemphigus vulgaris, pemphigus foliaceus as well as sera without serum autoantibodies with an agreement coefficient Cohen's κ between 0.88 and 0.97 [9]. More specifically, in 425 (93.6 %) of the 454 tested sera, the same result was obtained in both the routine multistep approach and the novel single step multivariant assay. In only 5 % of sera including patients with anti-laminin 332 mucous membrane pemphigoid, linear IgA disease, anti-p200 pemphigoid and epidermolysis bullosa acquisita, the routine procedures were advantageous. In the future, the extension of the

BIOCHIP™ mosaic and inclusion of additional target antigens such as laminin 332 and laminin γ1 will eliminate these short-comings. In fact, the NC1 domain of type VII collagen has meanwhile been integrated in the BIOCHIP™ mosaic showing a sensitivity of 91.8 % for epidermolysis bullosa acquisita sera and a specificity of 99.8 %, respectively [11].

Key Points

- The BIOCHIP™ mosaic shows a diagnostic accuracy comparable with the conventional multi-step approach.
- The highly standardized and easy to employ BIOCHIP™ mosaic may further facilitate the serological diagnosis of autoimmune blistering diseases.

References

1. Schmidt E, Zillikens D. Modern diagnosis of autoimmune blistering skin diseases. Autoimmun Rev. 2010;10:84–9.
2. Yoshida M, et al. Enzyme-linked immunosorbent assay using bacterial recombinant proteins of human BP230 as a diagnostic tool for bullous pemphigoid. J Dermatol Sci. 2006;41:21–30.
3. Ishii K, et al. Characterization of autoantibodies in pemphigus using antigen-specific enzyme-linked immunosorbent assays with baculovirus-expressed recombinant desmogleins. J Immunol. 1997;159:2010–7.
4. Sitaru C, et al. Enzyme-linked immunosorbent assay using multimers of the 16th non-collagenous domain of the BP180 antigen for sensitive and specific detection of pemphigoid autoantibodies. Exp Dermatol. 2007;16:770–7.
5. Schmidt E, et al. Novel ELISA systems for antibodies to desmoglein 1 and 3: correlation of disease activity with serum autoantibody levels in individual pemphigus patients. Exp Dermatol. 2010;19:458–63.
6. Probst C, et al. Development of ELISA for the specific determination of autoantibodies against envoplakin and periplakin in paraneoplastic pemphigus. Clin Chim Acta. 2009;410:13–8.

7. Saleh MA, et al. Development of NC1 and NC2 domains of type VII collagen ELISA for the diagnosis and analysis of the time course of epidermolysis bullosa acquisita patients. J Dermatol Sci. 2011;62:169–75.

8. Schmidt E, Zillikens D. Pemphigoid diseases. Lancet. 2013; 381:320–32.

9. van Beek N, et al. Serological diagnosis of autoimmune bullous skin diseases: prospective comparison of the BIOCHIP mosaic-based indirect immunofluorescence technique with the conventional multi-step single test strategy. Orphanet J Rare Dis. 2012;7:49.

10. Schmidt E, Zillikens D. Diagnosis and treatment of patients with autoimmune bullous disorders in Germany. Dermatol Clin. 2011;29:663–71.

11. Komorowski L, et al. Sensitive and specific assays for routine serological diagnosis of epidermolysis bullosa acquisita. J Am Acad Dermatol. 2013;68:e89–95.

Chapter 22
Desquamative Gingivitis Refractory to Conventional Treatments in a Young Female Desiring to Have a Child

Kristen Whitney and David Fivenson

A 29-year-old female presented with a 5 year history of pemphigus, characterized by recurrent painful sores in her mouth. She denied ever having lesions elsewhere on her body. Physical examination showed erosive or desquamative gingivitis of the upper and lower anterior and lateral gingival surfaces. Serologic studies revealed moderate to high anti-desmoglein 1 titers, ranging from 28 to 54 over the course of her disease, while anti-desmoglein three levels were always within normal limits. The patient was previously diagnosed with limited oral pemphigus based on routine histology, direct immunofluorescence findings and anti-desmoglein 1/3 ELISAs. Over the years, she had partial disease control with

K. Whitney, DO
Department of Dermatology,
St Joseph Mercy Health System,
Ann Arbor, MI, USA

D. Fivenson, M.D. (✉)
Dermatology, PLLC, Ann Arbor, MI, USA
e-mail: dfivenson@comcast.net

D.F. Murrell (ed.), *Clinical Cases in Autoimmune Blistering Diseases*, Clinical Cases in Dermatology 5, DOI 10.1007/978-3-319-10148-4_22, © Springer International Publishing Switzerland 2015

a variety of agents including: topical steroids, topical tacrolimus, topical dapsone and systemic prednisone, mycophenolate mofetil, and a combination of doxycycline + niacinamide. Hydroxychloroquine, dapsone and adalimumab were each tried for 3–6 months without efficacy. In addition to having recalcitrant pemphigus, she expressed interest in wanting to become pregnant.

Therapeutic Challenge: To find an efficacious medication that is safe during conception and pregnancy.

Based on the above case, which of the following medications would be a reasonable therapy in a female of childbearing age with resistant pemphigus who wants to get pregnant?

(A) Auranofin
(B) Methotrexate
(C) Azathioprine
(D) Cyclophosphamide

Answer: (A)

The patient was started on prednisone 20 mg/day and auranofin 3 mg three times daily combined with intermittent topical intraoral steroids for transient lesions. She had complete clearing of her oral erosions over 3 months and was tapered to 3–6 mg/day prednisone, subsequently conceived while on auranofin and continued on a dosage of auranofin 3 mg twice daily throughout her pregnancy. Desmoglein 1 antibodies ranged from 32 to 39 and desmoglein 3 antibodies remained negative during an uneventful pregnancy, resulting in a healthy, full-term baby. Approximately 9 months postpartum she began to flare despite increased oral steroids back to 20 mg/day and auranofin 3 mg three times daily. Desmoglein 1 antibody levels had risen to 49. She is currently tapering from high dose prednisone (1 mg/kg/day×4 weeks) and is considering rituximab and/or intravenous gamma globulin as she has completed her family planning and is not planning on any more children.

Diagnosis/Therapeutic Intervention

Pemphigus vulgaris limited to the oral mucosa, treated with auranofin.

Discussion

Pemphigus is a group of autoimmune blistering diseases in which the formation of intraepidermal blisters occur secondary to IgG autoantibodies against the cellular attachments of keratinocytes. Pemphigus can be broken down into three main subgroups: pemphigus vulgaris, pemphigus foliaceus and paraneoplastic pemphigus [2].

In pemphigus vulgaris (PV), the primary skin lesion is a flaccid, thin walled vesicle. Two subtypes of PV have been described: mucosal-dominant type in which the patient has autoantibodies against desmoglein 3, and the mucocutaneous type where antibodies against desmoglein 1 and 3 occur. All patients with pemphigus vulgaris develop oral lesions and over half of these patients will have cutaneous vesicles, bullae and erosions [2]. Our patient has a unique situation, in which she had relatively high titers of desmoglein 1 antibodies with consistently normal levels of desmoglein 3 antibodies, which would be serologically consistent with pemphigus foliaceus. Clinically however, she presented with and continues to have oral lesions only. Localized oral pemphigus vulgaris with anti-desmoglein 1 expression has been reported previously in the literature [4].

Systemic glucocorticoids are considered to be the first line treatment in PV. Steroid sparing agents are used for long-term disease management and include cytotoxic agents such as azathioprine, methotrexate, mycophenolate mofetil and cyclophosphamide. Noncytotoxic, steroid sparing agents are also used including tetracyclines + niacinamide, gold salts, dapsone [5], rituximab, infliximab [7] and adalimumab [10].

High dose steroids, the above mentioned cytotoxic agents and the tetracyclines are contraindicated in pregnancy, which limits the list of agents available for management of pregnant women to dapsone, hydroxychloroquine, low dose oral and topical steroids and gold [3]. Gold salts has been documented in the literature to be a safe and potential treatment in women of childbearing age with rheumatoid arthritis [1, 8].

Auranofin, the oral formulation of gold, has been reported as an option for steroid sparing therapy in patients with PV [9]. Roughly 25 % of auranofin is absorbed from the gastrointestinal tract and is excreted through the hepatobiliary tract. The half-life is estimated to be around 21 days. It is classified as a pregnancy category C.

Gold compounds have been shown to hinder both phagocytic and chemotactic properties of macrophages and polymorphonuclear leukocytes in vitro. In addition, it is believed that gold interferes with the complement cascade, affects prostaglandin synthesis, and inhibit lysosomal enzymes. There has been speculation that gold compounds are effective in pemphigus patients through either this interference with epidermal lysosomal enzymes, limiting blister formation, or thru effects on antigen presentation by dendritic cells [11].

Typical starting dose of auranofin is 3 mg twice daily, with a maximum dosage of 9 mg daily. It can take up to 6 months to achieve maximum efficacy, with most patients achieving a therapeutic response by 3–4 months. Common adverse effects with gold compounds include dermatitis, chelitis, stomatitis and diarrhea. Infrequently, proteinuria has been shown to occur in small percentage of patients, more commonly seen with parenteral gold, along with hematologic side effects consisting of leukopenia, thrombocytopenia, eosinophilia and rarely, aplastic anemia. There have been few reports of sudden onset of dyspnea progressing to pulmonary fibrosis [11]. All side effects reported are 75 % less frequent with oral formulations in compassion to parenteral gold salts [6]. To our knowledge there are no reports of adverse fetal outcomes at standard dosages of oral gold in humans, even though it can cross the placenta.

Key Points

- Pemphigus vulgaris is an autoimmune blistering disease subdivided into two types: mucosal-dominant and mucocutaneous, typically treated with high dose steroids and cytotoxic agents to suppress disease activity.
- Gold compounds, particularly auranofin, can be an effective steroid sparing treatment option in PV.
- Relative contraindications to gold compounds include renal or liver disease, inflammatory bowel disease, bone marrow suppression and prior gold-induced dermatitis.
- Auranofin, the oral formation of gold, is a FDA category C medication and allowed complete disease control for this patient during conception and pregnancy with no side effects to the mother or child.

References

1. Almarzougi M, Scarsbrook D, Klinkhoff A. Gold therapy in women planning pregnancy: outcomes in one center. J Rheumatol. 2007;34(9):1827–31.
2. Bolognia JL, Jorizzo JL, Schaffer JV. Dermatology. 3rd ed. Philadelphia, PA, USA: Elsevier; 2012.
3. Braunstein I, Werth V. Treatment of dermatologic connective tissue disease and autoimmune blistering disorders in pregnancy. Dermatol Ther. 2013;26(4):354–63.
4. Koga H, Ohyama B, Tsuruta D, et al. Five Japanese cases of antidesmoglein 1 antibody-positive and antidesmoglein 3 antibody-negative pemphigus with oral lesions. Br J Dermatol. 2012;166(5):976–80.
5. Mutasim DF. Management of autoimmune bullous diseases: pharmacology and therapeutics. J Am Acad Dermatol. 2004;51(6):859–77.
6. Papp KA, Shear NH. Systemic gold therapy. Clin Dermatol. 1991;9(4):535–51.
7. Perez OA, Patton T. Novel therapies for pemphigus vulgaris: an overview. Drugs Aging. 2009;26(10):833–46.
8. Tarp U, Graudal H. A followup study of children exposed to gold compounds in utero. Arthritis Rheum. 1985;28(2):235–6.

9. Thomas I. Gold therapy and its indications in dermatology. A review. J Am Acad Dermatol. 1987;16(4):845–54.
10. Vojackova N, Fialova J, Vanousova D, et al. Pemphigus vulgaris treated with adalimumab: case study. Dermatol Ther. 2012;25(1):95–7.
11. Wolverton S. Comprehensive dermatologic drug therapy. 3rd ed. Philadelphia, PA, USA: Elsevier; 2013.

CPSIA information can be obtained at www.ICGtesting.com
Printed in the USA
LVOW01s1316221114
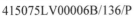
415075LV00006B/136/P